A NATIONAL ACADEMY OF MEDICINE
SPECIAL PUBLICATION

THE FUTURE OF HEALTH SERVICES RESEARCH

ADVANCING HEALTH SYSTEMS RESEARCH
AND PRACTICE IN THE UNITED STATES

Danielle Whicher, Kristin Rosengren, Sameer Siddiqi,
Lisa Simpson, *Editors*

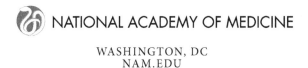

NATIONAL ACADEMY OF MEDICINE

WASHINGTON, DC
NAM.EDU

NATIONAL ACADEMY OF MEDICINE • 500 FIFTH STREET, NW • WASHINGTON, DC 20001

NOTICE: This publication has undergone peer review according to procedures established by the National Academy of Medicine (NAM). Publication by the NAM signifies that it is the product of a carefully considered process and is a contribution worthy of public attention, but it does not constitute endorsement of conclusions and recommendations by the NAM. The views presented in this publication are those of individual contributors and do not represent formal consensus positions of the authors' organizations; the NAM; or the National Academies of Sciences, Engineering, and Medicine.

Support for this publication was provided by AcademyHealth, American Association of Colleges of Nursing, American Board of Family Medicine, American Society of Anesthesiologists, Association of American Medical Colleges, and the Federation of American Hospitals. Support for this publication was also provided in part by the Robert Wood Johnson Foundation. The views expressed here do not necessarily reflect the views of the Foundation.

Library of Congress Cataloging-in-Publication Data

Names: Building the Evidence Base for Improving Health Care: Contributions, Opportunities, and Priorities (Workshop) (2018 : Washington, D.C.), author. | Whicher, Danielle, editor. | Rosengren, Kristin, editor. | Siddiqi, Sameer, editor. | Simpson, Lisa (Of AcademyHealth), editor.
Title: The future of health services research : advancing health systems research and practice in the United States / Danielle Whicher, Kristin Rosengren, Sameer Siddiqi, Lisa Simpson, editors.
Description: Washington, DC : National Academy of Medicine, [2018] | At head of title: A National Academy of Medicine special publication. | Includes bibliographical references.
Identifiers: LCCN 2018048491 (print) | LCCN 2018049191 (ebook) | ISBN 9781947103153 (E-book) | ISBN 9781947103146 (pbk. : alk. paper)
Subjects: | MESH: Health Services Research--methods | Health Services Research--trends | Research Design | Health Policy | United States | Congresses
Classification: LCC RA440.85 (ebook) | LCC RA440.85 (print) | NLM W 84.3 | DDC 362.1072--dc23
LC record available at https://lccn.loc.gov/2018048491

Suggested citation: Whicher, D., Rosengren, K., Siddiqi, S., Simpson, L., editors. 2018. *The Future of Health Services Research: Advancing Health Systems Research and Practice in the United States.* Washington, DC: National Academy of Medicine.

"Knowing is not enough; we must apply.
Willing is not enough; we must do."

—GOETHE

LEADERSHIP

IMPACT

for a healthier future

NATIONAL ACADEMY OF MEDICINE

ABOUT THE NATIONAL ACADEMY OF MEDICINE

The **National Academy of Medicine** is one of three Academies constituting the National Academies of Sciences, Engineering, and Medicine (the National Academies). The National Academies provide independent, objective analysis and advice to the nation and conduct other activities to solve complex problems and inform public policy decisions. The National Academies also encourage education and research, recognize outstanding contributions to knowledge, and increase public understanding in matters of science, engineering, and medicine.

The **National Academy of Sciences** was established in 1863 by an Act of Congress, signed by President Lincoln, as a private, nongovernmental institution to advise the nation on issues related to science and technology. Members are elected by their peers for outstanding contributions to research. Dr. Marcia McNutt is president.

The **National Academy of Engineering** was established in 1964 under the charter of the National Academy of Sciences to bring the practices of engineering to advising the nation. Members are elected by their peers for extraordinary contributions to engineering. Dr. C. D. Mote, Jr., is president.

The **National Academy of Medicine** (formerly the Institute of Medicine) was established in 1970 under the charter of the National Academy of Sciences to advise the nation on issues of health, health care, and biomedical science and technology. Members are elected by their peers for distinguished contributions to medicine and health. Dr. Victor J. Dzau is president.

Learn more about the National Academy of Medicine at NAM.edu.

PLANNING COMMITTEE ON BUILDING THE EVIDENCE BASE FOR IMPROVING HEALTH CARE

ANDREW BINDMAN, University of California San Francisco
CAROLYN CLANCY, US Department of Veterans Affairs
ELLIE DEHONEY, Research!America
ADAEZE ENEKWECHI, McDermott+Consulting
LEE FLEISHER, University of Pennsylvania
SHERRY GLIED, New York University
ATUL GROVER, Association of American Medical Colleges
SANDRA R. HERNÁNDEZ, California Health Care Foundation
CHARLES N. KAHN III, Federation of American Hospitals
GOPAL KHANNA, Agency for Healthcare Research and Quality
SUZANNE MIYAMOTO, American Association of Colleges of Nursing
ROBERT PHILLIPS, American Board of Family Medicine
ALONZO PLOUGH, Robert Wood Johnson Foundation
JOE V. SELBY, Patient Centered Outcomes Research Institute
LISA SIMPSON, AcademyHealth

NAM Staff

Development of this publication was facilitated by contributions of the following NAM staff, under the guidance of J. Michael McGinnis, NAM Leonard D. Schaeffer Executive Officer and Executive Director of the Leadership Consortium for a Value & Science-Driven Health System:

DANIELLE WHICHER, Senior Program Officer
MICHELLE JOHNSTON-FLEECE, Senior Program Officer (until September 2018)
HENRIETTA OSEI-ANTO, Senior Program Officer
SAMEER SIDDIQI, Technical Consultant
GWENDOLYN HUGHES, Senior Program Assistant (until July 2018)
JENNA OGILVIE, Communications Officer

AcademyHealth Staff

LISA SIMPSON, President and CEO
KRISTIN ROSENGREN, Vice President, Strategic Communications

Consultant

STEVE OLSON, Science Writer and Rapporteur

REVIEWERS

This publication was reviewed in draft form by individuals chosen for their diverse perspectives and technical expertise, in accordance with review procedures established by the NAM. We wish to thank the following individuals for their review of this publication:

ALEXANDER OMMAYA, Association of American Medical Colleges
ELEANOR M. PERFETTO, National Health Council
MEREDITH ROSENTHAL, Harvard T.H. Chan School of Public Health

Although the reviewers listed above provided many constructive comments and suggestions, they were not asked to endorse the content of the publication, nor did they see the final draft before it was published. Review of this publication was overseen by **Danielle Whicher,** Senior Program Officer, NAM and **J. Michael McGinnis,** Leonard D. Schaeffer Executive Officer, NAM. Responsibility for the final content of this publication rests entirely with the editors and the NAM.

FOREWORD

It is evident in multiple dimensions that health and health care in the United States is in a period of unprecedented opportunity, accompanied by very imposing challenges. The promises are clear. The biomedical and social sciences are providing new fundamental insights on sources and courses of disease and infirmity, along with new strategies for prevention, diagnosis, and treatment. Mapping the human genome has opened the door to better targeting of individual and public health interventions. Engineering technologies applicable from the nano- to macro- scale hold prospects for restructuring health and safety as integral products of our physical and biologic environments. Diagnostic and therapeutic interventions previously developed for delivery in sophisticated medical centers now have variations in development for delivery and use in remote settings. Data gathered with greater convenience to patients and families and delivered securely to a skilled site for interpretation and application offer prospects for both accelerated access to effectively tailored interventions and for continuous learning and improvement facilitated by artificial intelligence and machine learning. Advances of these sorts have yielded real gains for Americans: saving lives, extending life spans, and introducing progress against many chronic conditions, infectious diseases, and injuries. Similarly, meaningful contributions have been made to cost sharing, quality improvement, payment models, and patient safety.

Yet significant unmet challenges remain, and some of them are worsening. Health care costs in the United States still rank highest in the world, well above the next most expensive delivery system, now approaching 18% of the US Gross Domestic Product. Despite the magnitude of national spending, unacceptable disparities still exist in the health experiences of different population groups, and, for certain groups, those disparities are increasing to the point that life spans are actually decreasing. These persistent disparities are in part the product of lifelong inequities experienced by some groups, and in part the product of a longstanding divide between the delivery of health services and the access to social services—such as food, housing, and transportation—needed particularly in the context of the health risks in play.

Our payment systems remain substantially focused on rewarding service volume over value or outcomes. Further, the implications of environmental warming trends for treatment and prevention services and programs are poorly understood.

One thing is certainly clear: effective action to take full advantage of opportunities or to counter growing threats requires a timely, reliable, and continuously improving evidence base to guide decisions. Whether those decision-makers are clinicians, patients and families, executives from health care organizations, public health agencies, employers, or health payers or purchasers, they need to know what problems are in play and what works best, for whom, and under what circumstances. In the past, this has underscored the importance of health services research. Yet, ironically, at a time when the need is becoming more complex and more acute, when our realization of the importance of linking what happens inside clinic doors with what happens outside them, the support for health services research is softening. Especially needed at this time is a deepened capacity and commitment with a broader vision—one of a transformed capability for health systems research and practice embedded in health related initiatives throughout the nation.

Against this backdrop, a discussion among leaders and stakeholders in the field of health services research was convened in early 2018 by the National Academy of Medicine, with the partnership, support, and leadership of AcademyHealth, the American Association of Colleges of Nursing, the American Board of Family Medicine, the American Society of Anesthesiologists, the Association of American Medical Colleges, the Federation of American Hospitals, and the Robert Wood Johnson Foundation. It was a meeting planned by a steering group comprised of experts representing those fields, and bringing together many of the individuals and organizations that have helped to create, expand, and lead the field of health services research. Those gathered explored the broad terrain of the field, including its evolution, past accomplishments, emerging issues and tools, priorities for attention, and potential impact on health, health care, health costs, and individual and community engagement.

The discussion identified a number of priority topics, including development of more effective approaches for integrating data on social determinants with other health care data; determining which quality measures and outcomes are critical to improving patient-centered care; embedding research skills and tools in care delivery; developing models of patient and stakeholder engagement throughout the research process; understanding the impact on population health of alternative payment models, of innovative care delivery models, and of artificial intelligence in health care; building upon existing progress in patient safety and errors, and exploring how to best translate health services research and scale its impact within policy settings and health systems.

In assessing the historical pattern of public and private support for health services research, and the scope, scale, structure, and function of that support, observers suggested that perhaps as important as the topics identified for priority attention are the vision and strategies for engaging key stakeholders. Specifically, success in deepening the commitment and support base for the field will be advanced by the extent to which collaborative efforts using systems perspectives help foster a culture of continuous learning, development of the data infrastructure and research teams for real-time insights, gathering and communicating the contributions in personal, societal, and economic terms, and linking those returns to stakeholder investments.

Both the National Academy of Medicine and the Commonwealth Fund are committed to helping advance, expand, and deepen progress in the research field most central to generating better guidance for progress in the nation's health and health care. If the promise discussed here is a reliable harbinger of the prospects reported in *The Future of Health Services Research: Advancing Health Systems Research and Practice in the United States*, and if the requisite commitment is made to a sustained and well-networked public-private resource base for the accelerated health systems research envisioned, then the cost, quality, safety, outcome, and equity shortfalls that have for decades eluded solution, might instead see a quickening pace on the path to better health for all Americans.

J. Michael McGinnis, MD, MPP
Leonard Schaeffer Executive Officer
National Academy of Medicine

David Blumenthal, MD, MPP
President
The Commonwealth Fund

ACKNOWLEDGMENTS

The NAM would like to acknowledge and express its gratitude to those who participated in planning the symposium and developing this Special Publication.

First, we would like to thank the sponsors of this symposium and Special Publication: AcademyHealth, American Association of Colleges of Nursing, American Board of Family Medicine, American Society of Anesthesiologists, Association of American Medical Colleges, Federation of American Hospitals, and the Robert Wood Johnson Foundation, for their financial support. We would also like to thank members of the planning committee for their contributions in developing the symposium agenda and corresponding Special Publication.

This Special Publication was informed by presentations and discussions at a National Academy of Medicine Symposium on February 26-27, 2018, in Washington, DC, entitled *Building the Evidence Base for Improving Health Care: Contributions, Opportunities, and Priorities.*

A number of NAM staff played instrumental roles in coordinating the symposium and the preparing of this Special Publication, including Danielle Whicher, Michelle Johnston-Fleece, Henrietta Osei-Anto, Sameer Siddiqi, Gwendolyn Hughes, and Jenna Ogilvie. We would also like to acknowledge AcademyHealth for their participation in preparing this Special Publication, particularly Lisa Simpson and Kristin Rosengren. Additionally, we would like to thank Tammy Chang of the University of Michigan Medical School, Sean Lucan of the Albert Einstein College of Medicine, and Caroline Hagedorn of the National Institutes of Health for their insight and contributions. We would also like to thank Steve Olson for distilling key points from the symposium and assisting in the development of the manuscript. Finally, we would like to acknowledge the guidance and contributions of J. Michael McGinnis, Leonard D. Schaeffer Executive Officer and Executive Director of the Leadership Consortium for a Value & Science-Driven Health System.

CONTENTS

BOXES, FIGURES, AND TABLES

ACRONYMS AND ABBREVIATIONS

AARP	American Association of Retired Persons
AHRQ	Agency for Healthcare Research and Quality
APCD	All Payer Claims Databases
AQC	Alternative Quality Contract
CDC	United States Centers for Disease Control and Prevention
CMMI	Center for Medicare & Medicaid Innovation
CMS	Centers for Medicare & Medicaid Services
CPOE	Computerized Provider Order Entry
DOD	United States Department of Defense
EHR	Electronic Health Record
FDA	United States Food and Drug Administration
HCCI	Health Care Cost Institute
HCUP	Healthcare Cost and Utilization Project
HIPAA	Health Insurance Portability and Accountability Act
HSR&D	Health Services Research and Development Service
IOM	Institute of Medicine (now the National Academy of Medicine)
JAMA	Journal of the American Medical Association
MCPS	Medicare Claims Processing System
MEPS	Medical Expenditure Panel Survey
NAM	National Academy of Medicine
NHLBI	National Heart, Lung, and Blood Institute
NIH	National Institutes of Health

OECD   Organisation for Economic Co-operation and Development

PCORI   Patient-Centered Outcomes Research Institute
PCORnet   National Patient-Centered Clinical Research Network

RWJF   Robert Wood Johnson Foundation

SES   Socioeconomic Status

VA   United States Department of Veterans Affairs

SUMMARY

Health services research provides the foundation for progress, effectiveness, and value in health care. Given the widening gap between what should be possible and what is achieved in health and health care, strengthening the pillars of the nation's capacity to assess and improve health system performance is essential.

This was an oft-repeated observation at the National Academy of Medicine (NAM) workshop in February 2018 in Washington, DC, on *Building the Evidence Base for Improving Health Care: Contributions, Opportunities, and Priorities*. The workshop was sponsored by AcademyHealth, the American Association of Colleges of Nursing, the American Board of Family Medicine, the American Society of Anesthesiologists, the Association of American Medical Colleges, the Federation of American Hospitals, and the Robert Wood Johnson Foundation. Over the course of the day-and-a-half-long meeting, the participants examined funding trends, the federal and nonfederal organizations supporting health services research, the major contributions of the field, key future directions and priorities from the perspective of multiple stakeholders, and strategies for improving the ability of the field to address those priorities over the next decade.

Building on a historic base of certain path-breaking insight on how care delivery alters results, assessment of health services emerged as a field in the 1960s when federally-funded support for health care and construction of health care facilities grew rapidly, and has played a pivotal role in contributing to health policy and the delivery of health care services in the US. However, in the current policy environment, questions have been raised about the scope, scale, structure, and function of government support for health services research and, as a result, now is a critical time for the field to reflect on its past accomplishments; identify shortfalls, challenges, and future priorities; and investigate ways of organizing to effectively and efficiently address those challenges and priorities.

Current funding for health services research represents a very small percent of total research and development spending and of spending on health care in the US (0.3 percent) (Moses et al. 2015). Further, the number of projects supported by the top funders of health services research dropped overall from 2005 to 2011. Federal funding for health services research is provided by several different agencies, each with its own goals, and amounted to about $2.5 billion in Fiscal Year 2017 (U.S. Department of Health and Human Services, 2017). These agencies include the Agency for Healthcare Research and Quality, Centers for Disease Control and Prevention, Centers for Medicare and Medicaid Services, Health Resources and Services Administration, National Institutes of Health, and Veterans Health Administration. Additionally, although not a federal agency, the Patient-Centered Outcomes Research Institute also supports health services research. While these agencies do interact in a number of ways with each other and with other agencies not represented at the meeting, including the US Departments of Housing and Urban Development, Transportation, and Labor and Commerce, there continue to be opportunities to further coordinate efforts. Outside of the federal government, a number of private foundations support health services research, including the Robert Wood Johnson Foundation, the Peterson Center on Healthcare, the Commonwealth Fund, the California Health Care Foundation, and the Blue Shield of California Foundation, among others. In addition to coordinating efforts among federal agencies, it is important to consider how to best coordinate efforts between federal agencies and private foundations.

Federal and nonfederal funding for health services research has supported a number of efforts that have had a significant impact on health care policy and the way health systems operate in areas such as cost sharing, quality improvement, payment models, and patient safety. However, health services research has been less influential in informing more nuanced management and implementation decisions that health systems face. While there is value in conducting large multiyear research projects, timeliness matters. Participants underscored the need for efforts to focus on translation, communication, and implementation of results, as well as rapid cycle research projects that aim to inform policy makers and health systems leaders about issues they face as soon as is practical. Ultimately, this means developing capacity for health services research skills, techniques, and methods among operationally-focused teams within large health systems. Incentive structures should support this engagement with funding approaches that fit that purpose, and expand the research agenda to be more inclusive of short-term, policy-driven questions and practice-based studies.

In addition, there are a number of new tools and approaches that the field of health services research can leverage to contribute advances to care quality and efficiency, including developments in predictive analytics and artificial intelligence, large data resources such as National Patient-Centered Clinical Research Network (PCORNet), data standards, model data sharing agreements, and analysis tools. In addition, other developments include shared decision-making instruments and economic and incentive modeling approaches. Consideration of factors such as how health systems are organized, led, and reformed can improve the care that is delivered, ultimately leading to better outcomes for health care consumers. Health services researchers also continue to focus on bridging health and social services to improve access to care by addressing issues affecting access to care, including community factors, the availability of social services, and the social determinants of health. The importance of social determinants of health has been recognized for a number of years, and these factors can create a complex network of interlinked issues for health systems and researchers that require expanding the focus beyond academic health centers and hospitals to integrated primary care, community services, and public health. Within the health care system, access to care can be affected by insurance benefit designs that continually increase cost sharing. A key challenge for health services research is to determine which benefit design innovations decrease costs without having an adverse impact on health outcomes.

In order to leverage the new tools and approaches and incorporate additional data from community and other settings, it is critical to improve the national data infrastructure. Currently, cultural and political barriers, regulations, a lack of follow-through on public commitments to share data, legal challenges, and the growth of proprietary data, prohibit the sharing of data to improve health and health care. Moreover, the quality of most electronic health record and claims data is insufficient for supporting health services research and researchers often experience difficulty linking these data sources with each other, with data on relevant social factors, and with other patient-reported data. In addition to clinical and claims data, nationally representative surveys produce valuable high-quality data but many federally and state-supported surveys continue to be cut in response to budget pressures (Siddons, 2018). Policy levers for improving the data infrastructure and data sharing include developing data standards, uniform data systems across primary care settings, implementing policies to prevent data blocking and encourage truly interoperable systems, and developing additional guidance on the Health Insurance Portability and Accountability Act (HIPAA). However, a critical step to promote policy changes that might improve the data infrastructure and data access is illustrating how such changes might add value for end users in leveraging data to support research insights and health improvement.

While raising macro-level issues such as strategic coordination of research agendas and improving the national infrastructure for a fully interoperable health information system, participants emphasized various emerging strategic field focus priorities for the next decade, including:

- structured approaches to assessing, applying, and adapting the delivery system to insights and tools related to precision medicine;

- system strategies for ensuring patient safety in the face of an increasingly complex diagnostic and treatment environment;
- embedding health services research skills and tools into care delivery as a basic component of a continuously learning health system;
- establishing reliable data from the routine care experience as a secure utility enhancing evidence development, predictive modeling, and continuous care improvement;
- incorporating necessary demographic, environmental, social, and community data as an integral component of that data utility;
- devising and demonstrating the impact of innovative payment and care delivery models for improving system performance and population health;
- identification and application of quality assessment metrics that are most reliable at gauging system-wide performance in delivering care and improving health;
- positioning patient and family involvement, interests, priorities, and data as a central resource for care design and assessment;
- developing the full and effective use of artificial intelligence and machine learning as transformational resources for knowledge development and services improvement; and
- effective approaches to translating and scaling research insights, including effective expression of the consequences of inaction.

The range of the issues is so substantial that relying on spontaneous and sometimes serendipitous response capacity in the field will not meet the need. Rather, a deliberate and coordinated set of activities is required to prepare—to transform—the field. In effect, participants individually and collectively presented a call to action for the field to mobilize sustained initiatives to:

- expand the **vision** to account for the full range of health system forces in play;
- develop a robust taxonomy of the issue and leverage **priorities** for action;
- identify the **tools** and strategies—available and emerging—to refine and deploy in the change process;
- steward the societal-wide advancement of a **culture of continuous learning** and sharing throughout the system;
- foster the development of the **data infrastructure and research teams** required for real-time insights and feedback in the virtuous cycle of continuous learning;

- create a working **network** of stakeholders, including patients as partners in research, for expedited coordination, collaboration, and, as required, governance;
- establish shared network-wide **goals** and a process for tracking and adapting strategies;
- characterize the anticipated and actual **results** for improvement, in qualitative and quantitative personal, societal, and economic terms;
- **link** those real and potential returns to investments and investment requirements among stakeholders—federal and nonfederal; and
- capture and **communicate** the contributions, real and potential, in a broad, visible, and deliberate campaign.

In the final analysis, addressing the insights, opportunities, and obligations identified during this NAM meeting will require sustained and deliberate conversations involving stakeholders from throughout the nation. Those conversations have started, but achieving their potential for impact will require commitment and active involvement in the years ahead from the organizations represented at the meeting, not only on their own behalf, but also as recruiters, motivators, and engagers of public and private stakeholders across the nation. Congress has recently made resources available and delivered a mandate to study future federal funding in the field. This NAM meeting and publication can serve as a reference and foundation for that work, as the physical and financial health of the nation is at stake.

1

INTRODUCTION AND BACKGROUND

Health services research provides the foundation for progress, effectiveness, and value in health care. Given the widening gap between what should be possible and what is achieved in health and health care, strengthening the pillars of the nation's capacity to assess and improve health system performance is essential. For more than a half century, health services research has been poised to inform and guide decision-making in health and health care. Building on a historic base of certain path-breaking insight on how care delivery alters results, assessment of health services emerged as a field in the 1960s when federally-funded support for health care and construction of health care facilities grew rapidly, and has played a pivotal role in contributing to health policy and the delivery of health care services in the US. However, in the current policy environment, questions have been raised about the scope, scale, structure, and function of government support for health services research and, as a result, now is a critical time for the field to reflect on its past accomplishments; identify shortfalls, challenges, and future priorities; and investigate ways of organizing to effectively and efficiently address those challenges and priorities.

Health progress is shaped by advances in three dimensions: understanding the causes and processes of disease, disability, or injury (etiologies); developing approaches to ameliorate or eliminate the impact of those causes and processes (interventions); and determining the effectiveness, efficiency, and consequences of alternative interventions and strategies for their delivery (services). Health services research activities are anchored in the service delivery domain, but many of the analytic tools and findings are applicable to each, hence the overlap can be substantial (McGinnis, 2018).

Perhaps the first structured trial of alternative service intervention strategies demonstrates the bridging nature of etiologic, intervention, and service studies: the 1747 experiment by the Scottish naval physician James Lind, using empirically-based dietary approaches to reduce scurvy among sailors (Lind, 1753). Dividing the sailors into six groups receiving standard diets, and each supplemented by one variable element, he observed that those receiving lemons and limes fared significantly better, even though the basis was unknown and Vitamin C was not identified for more than 150 years.

In the medical care setting, the best known early example of health services research dates to the Hungarian physician Ignaz Semmelweis who, while providing obstetrical care in 1847 in the Vienna General Hospital, proposed routine hand-washing with a chlorinated lime solution after observing that maternal deaths from fever were several times higher on wards for physician deliveries, relative to those for midwife deliveries (Semmelweis, 1861, 1983 English translation). Semmelweis based his proposal on the observations 30 years earlier of A.G. Labarraque, a French chemist, that such a solution could prevent the spread of infection from animal processing facilities and morgues (Labarraque, 1829). It also set the stage for later statistical work on sanitation in medical care, advanced by Florence Nightingale, the British mathematician and nurse who systematically shaped the delivery and assessment of nursing.

Over the nineteenth and early twentieth centuries, as understanding grew regarding the sources and nature of the spread of many infectious diseases, as well as the identification of groups at higher social and environmental risk, so did mandates for the capacity to develop the data and records infrastructure for tracking and studying the spread and behavior of the disease. Health services research began to take shape as a field of scientific inquiry in the United States in the 1960s, when federally funded support for payment for health care and construction of health care facilities grew rapidly. With these increased investments, interest and support for their assessment grew, as did some federally sponsored data capacities to provide a needed infrastructure.

At that time a relatively small group of academic researchers developed key conceptual approaches to studying issues involving the cost, quality, and accessibility of health care (Bindman, 2013), but the numbers began to accelerate, catalyzed by the attention from both the public and private sectors. In 1968, following a 1967 Congressional authorization, the Department of Health, Education, and Welfare established the first National Center for Health Services Research & Development. Shortly thereafter, the Robert Wood Johnson Foundation, established in 1971, made health services research a primary emphasis of its grant-making and field development. Over the past five decades, a substantial field has developed that, while providing critical insights into the costs and quality of personal health services, is the central source of information and insights on how our health system functions as a whole. As will be considered throughout the descriptions in this publication of the historical roots and evolving foci, health services research now extends far beyond the delivery of individual health care to the assessment of how systems behave and interface to shape health status and outcomes.

The contributions of what we now call health services research have been of seminal importance to health progress on topics such as quality improvement and patient safety and in laying the groundwork for integrative progress in fields ranging from psychology and economics to pharmacoepidemiology, genetic counseling, and personalized medicine. Ironically, at a time in which appreciation has never been higher for both the need and potential from health services research, the political and financial support for sustenance and growth appear to be weakening. Although the 2018 Agency for Healthcare Research and Quality (AHRQ) appropriation increased by $10M since 2017, the AHRQ appropriation has declined by $37M since 2014 (Agency for Healthcare Research and Quality, 2018).

As the complexity of care and care delivery increases due to our aging population and the development of more intervention prospects, we need the capacity to embed effectiveness insights and evidence generation directly into the care delivery process. As the costs of care continue to increase beyond sustainability at both the institutional and societal levels, the need is for the real-time, rigorous assessment of costs and outcomes. In the face of the challenges and critical decision points, core stakeholders, with the vital interests of the nation in prominent focus, coordinated to convene a national meeting under the auspices of the National Academy of Medicine.

NATIONAL ACADEMY OF MEDICINE WORKSHOP

This publication presents a summary of the discussion at a meeting called for by the leaders of the field of health services research, planned by a steering group comprised of experts representing those field leaders, and sponsored by stakeholder organizations that have been its stewards—including AcademyHealth, the American Association of Colleges of Nursing, the American Board of Family Medicine, the American Society of Anesthesiologists, the Association of American Medical Colleges, the Federation of American Hospitals, and the Robert Wood Johnson Foundation. The impetus for the meeting was very much in the spirit of a field which, throughout its history, has engaged in study of its own internal dynamics and its relationships with the broader health care community and policy makers (Westfall et al. 2007, Pittman, 2010; Gold, 2016). Within the National Academy of Medicine (NAM), the NAM Leadership Consortium for a Value & Science-Driven Health System provided the coordinating capacity for planning and implementing the workshop, entitled *Building the Evidence Base for Improving Health Care: Contributions, Opportunities, and Priorities* and held on February 26-27, 2018, at the National Academy of Sciences Building in Washington, DC.

BOX 1–1

Focus and Goals of the Workshop

FOCUS: Contributions of health services research to effectiveness and efficiency in health and health care, and key priorities for health services research as a means of generating the evidence required to guide transformative health and health care progress in the next two decades.

CORE QUESTIONS

1. **Contributions:** How has health services research contributed to improvement in health gains and health care access, delivery, and quality—at various levels: system, organization, practice, and health care interfaces?

2. **Priorities:** What are the challenges, opportunities, and priorities for health services research in the next decade and beyond for improving access, safety, quality, value, and patient/family engagement in a changing health care environment while reducing spending growth and advancing population health progress?

3. **Support:** What are the current public and private sources of support for health services research; what trends are in play; and do the metrics of decision-making and assessment vary by source and focus (e.g., technology assessment, clinical guidelines, care quality and safety, primary care, utilization and financing)? What should be the role of federal funding for health services research now and in the long-term?

4. **Organization:** How are health services research opportunities identified? How is health services research funded, coordinated, and results disseminated? How might these processes be improved? What is or should be the profile of a governance structure for health services research?

5. **Statutory mandate:** What might be the consequences given current legislative mandates related to priorities? How might important emphases be sustained and nurtured?

INTENDED OUTCOMES: Identify unique opportunities for the field of health services research to advance rigorous, timely, and relevant evidence and to inform national progress toward a health system that is person-centered, high-performing, and continuously learning.

SOURCE: National Academy of Medicine, 2018.

The meeting brought together many of the individuals and organizations that have helped to create, expand, and lead the field of health services research. Workshop presenters and other participants included a balanced and geographically diverse representation of evidence producers, evidence users, and funders of health services research from across the United States to ensure diverse perspectives. Appendix A contains the workshop participant list.

The workshop was designed to acknowledge the past accomplishments of health services research; identify shortfalls, challenges, and future priorities for the field; and investigate ways of organizing the field to address those challenges and future priorities. (Appendix B contains the workshop agenda.) It sought to reexamine the vision for health services research while also engaging in reality testing of the expectations and current status of the field. Box 1-1 presents the focus of the meeting, the core questions it was designed to answer, and the meeting's intended outcomes.

POLICY CONTEXT

Opening remarks from the NAM and AcademyHealth, representing key organizers of this workshop, emphasized the discussion's timeliness. In the current changing health care environment, the contributions of health services research have never been more important, NAM President Victor Dzau observed. Existing evidence needs to be widely implemented; the areas in greatest need of new evidence need to be identified; a strong data infrastructure needs to be built; critical issues such as the social determinants of health need to be investigated; the link between primary care and social and community services needs to be explored; and innovations in consumer-driven care and tiered networks need to be examined. Dzau pointed out that transformative approaches to improve patient and physician experiences and outcomes also need to be considered while the current fee-for-service system are giving way to population- and value-based payment models that change provider incentives. Novel data analytics are needed to target and improve care, reduce waste, improve patient outcomes, and yield innovations in evaluating cost and care.

Health services researchers, by studying the quality, accessibility, cost, and outcomes of health care, deliver the information for health care providers, insurers, government, and patients to assist in making the right decisions for better care. But Dzau also pointed to a worrisome softening of the support base, with, for example, the Administration's fiscal year 2018 budget proposing folding the Agency for Healthcare Research and Quality (AHRQ) under the National Institutes of Health (NIH), which, if it led to reductions in both funds and priority for the field "could deal a significant blow to the field of health services research." Although Congress rejected this proposal and continued supporting AHRQ in its current state, a similar proposal was included in the 2019 budget. In concluding his comments, Dzau underscored the importance of working with the federal government, as well as with private philanthropies, to sustain the funding leadership necessary for the field.

Building on these themes, Lisa Simpson, President of AcademyHealth, observed that health services research is at an inflection point, with questions being raised about the scope, scale, structure, and function of government support for health services research. "Our shared mission requires a sustained and sustainable federal investment in health services research and data," she said, "but, as in other areas of federal support, money is necessary . . . but not sufficient. We also need a functional and efficient structure for federally funded health services research that delivers on its promise of advancing knowledge, informing choices, and improving health and health care."

Simpson evoked three broad principles from AcademyHealth. First, evidence is essential. The policies and practices affecting health and the performance of the health system should be informed by the best and most relevant evidence. What works for whom in what context? How can the answers be implemented at scale to achieve better health and better health care?

Second, the production of evidence should be a public good, and the development of the health services research workforce and a high-quality data and information infrastructure should be part of the overall federal investment in health research. Simpson noted that "Yes, the private sector needs to be at the table. But if all the evidence is created behind proprietary walls, what will happen? Relying purely on market forces for improvement is likely to perpetuate and deepen the very real disparities and inequities that we have in this country."

Third, diverse perspectives lead to richer and more nuanced understanding of issues related to health and the performance of the health system. That is one of the reasons why this workshop is so valuable—because the diversity of views represented provide very important input to the continuing conversation. Simpson indicated that it is now time to step back and take a broader look at the federal infrastructure to push ourselves to assess whether and how we will be able to meet the data and evidence needs of policy makers, health care system leaders, patients, consumers, and communities now and in the future.

Finally, as J. Michael McGinnis, NAM Leonard D. Schaeffer Executive Officer, also said in his opening remarks, now is a time "in which our tools and knowledge for application in health and health care have never been greater, in which expenditures have never been higher, and in which the gap between our accomplishments and our potential has never been clearer." Perhaps the most pressing policy context relates to the economic unsustainability of the growth in health care costs, and relatedly, the inability to identify ways in which the nation can find effective ways of bridging what happens inside clinic doors to what happens outside that ultimately determines the value of our investment. Given that context, "we've gathered here to discuss solutions—and the science of bringing solutions to practice is through health services research."

ORGANIZATION AND THEMES

The flow of this summary publication follows the meeting structure. Chapter 1 presents the introductory context, and chapter 2 examines the history, funding environment, and status of health services research. Since its formation in the 1960s, health services research has expanded substantially, but it still faces some of the same issues it faced early in its history. Many parts of the federal government fund health services research, but they typically ask different types of questions, and coordination among agencies is sometimes lacking. Foundations also have played an important role in supporting the field, again with a wide range of research interests.

Chapter 3 looks at the impact of health services research on decisions ranging from macro-level policy choices to micro-level implementation decisions. Health services research has made transformative contributions on multiple levels. For example, health services research has improved detection and minimization of health care mistakes in key clinical circumstances, led to the development of patient safety indicators, and informed national policy conversations. However, while health services research has been particularly impactful in motivating the policy changes mentioned, it has had more limited utility in defining service delivery changes that clearly demonstrate improved value—in part because these changes often require broader systemic and cultural reward system changes to be implemented and sustained, and partly because of a mismatch between traditional academic reward structures and the institutional reward systems involved in moving new knowledge to practice.

Chapter 4 considers emerging issues and approaches important to engage in better guiding health system performance. For example, predictive modeling and artificial intelligence have made it possible to target interventions to the people who are most likely to become high-need, high-cost patients. In addition, new ways of organizing, leading, and reforming health care systems, including large-scale culture change and alternative payment models, can lead to better quality and outcomes while slowing the rate of growth in health care spending.

Chapter 5 examines emerging approaches to improving access to care and bridging health and social services. Ubiquitous forces shape the health of populations, though their effects are difficult to separate out in studies of health problems. Health services research could accelerate its evolving focus of attention beyond academic health centers and hospitals to integrated primary care, community health services, and public health. In the process, it could provide valuable new knowledge on benefits design, caring for patients with complex health needs, and the continuum and coordination of care.

Chapter 6 turns to the data infrastructure for health services research and related quality and care improvement activities. Large amounts of health care data exist and have been used by health services researchers, but many data still are unstructured and/or controlled by others and unavailable to researchers. Challenges include proprietary barriers, the sustainability of data sources, and the dissemination of data and the results derived from data. In addition, the currently available data have serious limitations and are often expensive to access. Novel analytic approaches and innovative data-gathering techniques (such as the use of smart phones) bear significant promise.

Chapter 7 draws on earlier discussions to describe potential research and infrastructure priorities for health services research. Priorities for the field of health services research are considered through the lenses of different stakeholders, including policy makers, clinicians, patient advocates, and payers. The discussion highlighted the importance of additional research on health care financing and the impact on patients, high-need patients, patient preferences regarding data sharing, provider burnout, provider consolidation, and understanding the social determinants of health.

Chapter 8 loops back across key points to identify appropriate mechanisms for organizing the field of health services research in the twenty-first century. A research agenda for the twenty-first century would include not only research topics but how that research will be applied, which constituents are involved, and the value proposition for each constituency. Shared goals could foster public investment in innovation, evaluation, and implementation of what is learned, and a governing structure for investments in health services research could help ensure that decisions are made in an efficient and coherent manner. In addition, the field needs to develop a communication strategy that articulates its value in terms of improving health, health care, and health policy. Transforming health services research will require ongoing involvement from the organizations represented at the meeting, not only on their own behalf, but as recruiters, motivators, and engagers of public and private stakeholders across the nation.

2

HEALTH SERVICES RESEARCH ECOSYSTEM

Health services is continuously evolving, in concept and practice. In 1979, a National Academy of Medicine (then Institute of Medicine [IOM]) committee defined health services research as "inquiry to produce knowledge about the structure, processes, or effects of personal health services" (IOM, 1979). Since then, as noted in chapter 1, the purview of health services research has substantially broadened, and AcademyHealth, the professional organization devoted specifically to engaging health services researchers, now draws on a description defining health services research as "the multidisciplinary field of scientific investigation that studies how social factors, financing systems, organizational structures and processes, health technologies, and personal behaviors affect access to health care, the quality and cost of health care, and ultimately our health and well-being." (Lohr and Steinwachs, 2002). In other words, understanding the systemic factors in play, and how they impact health and health care throughout institutional and uniquely personal forces, has substantially broadened the necessary analytic terrain. At several points during the workshop, presenters and participants discussed the concepts, history, development, and funding of health services research since its origins. Elements of those discussions are combined and summarized here, along with a broad overview of the related interests and activities of federal agencies and other funders that support health services research, and observations on how those funding agencies interact with one another.

HISTORY AND FUNDING OF THE FIELD

Health services research began to emerge as a formal and distinct field in the 1960s as investments in personal health services began to expand, leading President Johnson to propose legislation to establish the National Center for Health Services Research and Development in 1967, noting that attainment of national health care objectives and efficient management of the federal government's disparate research activities required a coordinated effort. When questions arose about the relevance of health services research to the needs of decision makers, the White House Office of Science and Technology Policy commissioned an IOM study published in 1979 that called for greater coordination across the federal government and for a greater proportion of funding to go to investigator-initiated extramural research (IOM, 1979).

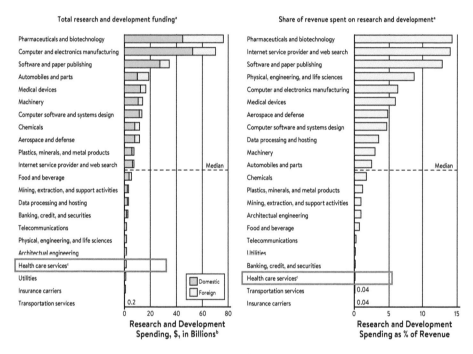

FIGURE 2-1 | Health care services represent a small share of industrial research-and-development funding (left) and percentage of revenues spent on research and development (right) by US-based companies

SOURCE: Moses et al. 2015

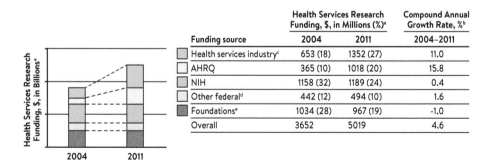

	Health Services Research Funding, $, in Millions (%)[a]		Compound Annual Growth Rate, %[b]
Funding source	2004	2011	2004–2011
Health services industry[c]	653 (18)	1352 (27)	11.0
AHRQ	365 (10)	1018 (20)	15.8
NIH	1158 (32)	1189 (24)	0.4
Other federal[d]	442 (12)	494 (10)	1.6
Foundations[e]	1034 (28)	967 (19)	-1.0
Overall	3652	5019	4.6

FIGURE 2-2 | US funding for health-services research grew from 2004 to 2011

SOURCE: Simpson, 2018

AGENCY	FY2010	FY2011	FY2012	FY2013	FY2014	FY2015	FY2016	FY2017
Agency for Healthcare Research and Quality	$397.00	$384.00	$405.00	$433.00	$464.00	$465.00	$427.60	$416.60
Base Discretionary		$372.00	$372.00	$369.00	$364.00	$364.00	$334.00	$324.00
Prevention and Public Health Fund		$12.00	$12.00	$6.00	$7.00			
Patient-Centered Outcomes Research Fund		$8.00	$24.00	$57.50	$93.00	$101.00	$93.60	$92.15
CDC: National Centers for Health Statistics	$138.70	$168.00	$168.00	$168.00	$153.90	$155.40	$160.40	$160.40
Base Discretionary	$138.70	$138.00	$138.00	$138.00	$153.90	$155.40	$160.40	$160.40
Prevention and Public Health Fund		$30.00	$30.00	$30.00				
CDC: Public Health Research/PHSSR	$31.20	$21.00	$	$	$	$	$	$
Base Discretionary		$11.00						
Prevention and Public Health Fund		$10.00						
CDC: Prevention Research Centers	$33.70	$28.00	$28.00	$23.40	$25.50	$25.50	$25.50	$25.50
Base Discretionary		$18.00	$18.00	$8.10	$25.50	$25.50	$25.50	$25.50
Prevention and Public Health Fund		$10.00	$10.00	$15.30				
CMS: Research, Demonstration & Evaluation Projects	$36.00	$35.00	$21.20	$20.10	$20.10	$20.10	$20.10	$20.10
HRSA: Rural Health Policy Development	$10.00	$9.90	$10.00	$9.30	$9.40	$9.40	$9.40	$9.40
National Institutes of Health*	$1,131.00	$1,116.00	$1,164.00	$1,262.00	$1,342.00	$1,437.00	$1,692.00	$1,770.00
Veterans Health Administration	$84.00	$91.30	$90.00	$90.30	$96.00	$91.30	$97.80	$104.60
PCORI	$50.00	$120.00	$161.60	$240.70	$425.70	$422.50	$471.00	$466.10
TOTAL (PROGRAM LEVEL)	$1,912.00	$1,973.00	$1,958.00	$2,241.00	$2,536.00	$2,627.00	$2,904.00	$2,972.70

*NIH Estimates of Funding for Various Research, Condition, and Disease Categories (RCDC). https://report.nih.gov/categorical_spending.aspx. Based on official federal agency budgets. SOURCE: Simpson et al, 2018 [Pending Citation]

FIGURE 2-3 | Federal funding for health services research grew from 2010 to 2017. SOURCE: Simpson, 2018

	2005	2007	2009	2011	2013	2015	2016	CHANGE (%) BETWEEN 2005 AND 2016
National Institutes of Health (combined)	630	561	845	619	630	513	586	-6.98
Robert Wood Johnson Foundation (RWJF)	339	294	189	138	130	68	51	-84.9
Agency for Healthcare Research and Quality (AHRQ)	122	186	206	140	243	232	245	100.8
Centers for Medicare and Medicaid Services (CMS)	95	31	22	11	13	8	12	-87.4
Health Resources and Services Administration (HRSA), Office of Rural Health Policy	81	22	27	20	28	27	8	-90.1
Department of Veterans Affairs (VA)	68	101	187	167	178	105	87	27.9
Patient-Centered Outcomes Research Institute (PCORI)	-	-	-	-	136	117	117	-14.0
Commonwealth Fund	50	100	42	112	38	61	-	26.0
Total	1385	1295	1518	1207	1396	1131	1106	-20.14

Based on data from the US National Library of Medicine's Health Services Research Projects (HSRProj) in Progress

FIGURE 2-4 | The number of projects supported by top funders dropped from 2005 to 2016
SOURCE: Simpson, 2018

Lisa Simpson, president and chief executive officer of AcademyHealth, noted that although funding for health services research has grown, it remains a very small percentage of total spending on health care (0.3 percent) (Figure 2-1). The total funding for health services research, as calculated by Moses et al. (2015), increased from 2004 to 2011 (the last date covered in the analysis) and, in that year, exceeded $5 billion (Figure 2-2), with a boost in 2011 because of federal funds being spent to recover from the recession under the American Recovery and Reinvestment Act.

A number of federal agencies, each with its own goals, fund health services research. Together, this funding amounted to about $2.5 billion in Fiscal Year 2017, with approximately two-thirds of that from the NIH (Figure 2-3). As a result of this funding distribution, NIH-funded research, with its particular emphasis on investigator-initiated academic research, provides incentives that heavily influence health services research. Simpson also pointed out that the

Department of Defense (DOD) is not included in this total because of the difficulty of separating out its funding, but DOD funds health services research and, Simpson stated, is "interested in doing more."

Simpson also reported specifically on funding for AHRQ, which was established in 1989 as the Agency for Health Care Policy and Research and acquired its current name during a 1999 reauthorization. AHRQ funding has increased from approximately $173 million in 1999 to $381 million in 2012, according to an analysis of an appropriations conference report by the Association of American Medical Colleges. This represented 0.68 percent of total Public Health Service funding in 1999 and 0.83 percent of the total in 2012. However, Simpson also noted that AHRQ has not been reauthorized and the president's recent budget submission proposed reorganizing the agency into a National Institute for Research on Safety and Quality as part of the NIH. Another element of uncertainty for the field is the decline in the number of projects supported by top funders, which dropped overall from 2005 to 2016 (Figure 2-4). Though some projects have become bigger, the overall numbers reveal a significant reduction in the number of projects in health services research which are funded.

PHILANTHROPIC LEADERSHIP

Many private foundations support health services research, including organizations such as the Robert Wood Johnson Foundation (RWJF), the Peterson Center on Healthcare, the Commonwealth Fund, the California Healthcare Foundation, and the Blue Shield of California Foundation, among many others. Richard Besser, president and chief executive officer of RWJF, commented on the role of foundations in supporting health services research. RWJF "has spent four decades helping to develop a generation of exceptional [health services] researchers who are dedicated to putting evidence to work in the rocky terrain of the real world," said Besser. "We have supported research and leadership development programs that take a multidisciplinary approach to the way care is organized, financed, delivered, and consumed." Most recently, a new set of research programs explore how other sectors such as education, criminal justice, housing, transportation, and agriculture influence health outcomes.

Besser highlighted several examples of research supported by RWJF that aim to improve the delivery, quality, cost, and coordination of health care. Recent research in Kentucky on Medicaid work requirements found that about 357,000 recipients who are currently not working could be affected by proposed policy changes. Nearly half of these people are more than 50 years old, a quarter do not have a high school education, and three-quarters have a serious health limitation or no car or Internet access. This is "the kind of rapid turnaround health services research that is critically needed to help inform the policy debate," he said. "It doesn't mean that the policy debate will go in the direction that those of us in health would like it to go. But at least it can be informed with facts." Another example is health services research involving implementation and evaluation of the first locally designed and financed public health program for the Cheyenne River Sioux tribe in South Dakota. The research is using a community-based participatory research approach to elicit tribal preferences in designing and implementing the program. It is also examining the relationship that develops between state and federal agencies in meeting the tribe's needs. "We are hopeful that this kind of work will help inform the design of other health programs built to answer the wants and needs of specific communities."

Besser also underscored the importance for public and private cooperation and collaboration in building the evidence base to improve health and health care. The section below highlights the important roles of major federal agencies using and supporting the field.

AGENCY FOR HEALTHCARE RESEARCH AND QUALITY (AHRQ)

AHRQ's role is to focus on the health care system as a whole, said the agency's director, Gopal Khanna. It funds research and works with doctors, nurses, health systems, and others to foster the provision of safe, high-quality health care for all Americans. It tracks progress and gets information to those who need it quickly by synthesizing diffuse data points and turning them into usable information, thereby translating and operationalizing knowledge for end users. This means working with primary care providers, hospitals, and nursing homes to help them understand what works best and to operationalize innovations.

Though AHRQ is smaller than many other federal agencies, it collaborates with a variety of partners to leverage its capacities. It works with the Centers for Medicare and Medicaid Services (CMS) to support the Hospital Improvement Innovation Network and the Community-based Care Transitions Program.[1] It works with the Patient-Centered Outcomes Research Institute (PCORI) to disseminate and implement patient-centered outcomes research. It works with the Centers for Disease Control and Prevention (CDC) to combat health

---

1 More information about the Hospital Improvement Innovation Network and the Community-based Care Transitions Program is available at https://partnershipforpatients.cms.gov/about-the-partnership/hospital-engagement-networks/thehospitalengagementnetworks.html and https://innovation.cms.gov/initiatives/CCTP, respectively.

care-associated infections, and it does synthesis work with a variety of partners. "I'm eager to sustain and expand on these collaborative partnerships," Khanna said.

AHRQ's work falls into three categories: research and evidence, tools and training, and data and measures. It also has three priority areas that capture its goals: patient safety, practice, and data and insight. In the area of patient safety, AHRQ is well known for its achievements in the areas of health care–associated infections. It is also working on medical errors, antibiotic resistance, and diagnostic safety. In the area of practice, AHRQ is investing in implementation research and developing tools and resources that clinicians can use at the point of care. For example, its EvidenceNOW program is working with 1,500 small and medium-sized primary care practices to accelerate the use of evidence to improve heart health.[2] In the area of data and insight, AHRQ has developed data resources, such as the Healthcare Cost and Utilization Project (HCUP) and the Medical Expenditure Panel Survey (MEPS), to improve health care delivery.[3] It also develops statistical briefs on such high-priority topics as opioid use and misuse, mental health services, and childhood obesity, and it uses predictive analytics to identify problems and develop innovations.

AHRQ has an impact beyond its size, said Khanna, but more resources would mean more opportunities to expand its data resources and leverage its expertise. Additional funding also would provide more opportunities to operationalize innovations to get research disseminated and implemented in everyday practice. "Successful project implementation requires time and money to support infrastructure, tools, and participation," he said.

NATIONAL INSTITUTES OF HEALTH (NIH)

With 27 institutes and centers, NIH has a two-pronged mission, reported George Mensah, director of the Center for Translation Research and Implementation Science at the National Heart, Lung, and Blood Institute: 1) to advance basic science; and 2) to advance human health. The tag line for NIH is "turning discovery into health," and, Mensah observed, "fundamental discoveries cannot be turned into health without a focus on health services research."

NIH is the primary federal funder of basic, clinical, and translational medical research. As an essential component of this investment, NIH supports health services research to understand how to best translate research findings into

---

2   More information about EvidenceNOW is available at https://www.ahrq.gov/evidencenow/index.html.

3   More information about HCUP and MEPS is available at https://www.ahrq.gov/research/data/hcup/index.html and https://meps.ahrq.gov/mepsweb, respectively.

evidence that informs medical practice. NIH-supported health services research generally builds upon categorical (e.g., aging) or disease-specific (e.g., HIV/AIDS, cancer) research related to the missions of individual NIH Institutes and Centers, and includes investigator-initiated research as well as targeted research in response to specific funding opportunity announcements. Health services research projects supported by NIH focus on moving NIH-supported clinical and translational discoveries into routine clinical practice, ultimately improving health outcomes.

NIH Institutes and Centers support a broad portfolio of health services research projects, which aim to promote more effective and efficient means of prevention, screening, and treatment, and reduce health disparities by addressing the needs of all populations. The agency also funds the development and maintenance of infrastructure and resources to facilitate health services research, and to enable the dissemination and implementation of health services research findings. The NIH Health Systems Research Collaboratory is an example of a focused NIH-wide investment to develop infrastructure for health services research; specifically, to strengthen the national capacity to implement cost-effective, large-scale research studies that involve health care delivery organizations. As one measure of its commitment to health services research, the National Heart, Lung, and Blood Institute set up the Center for Translation Research and Implementation Science.[4]

NIH also coordinates with other federal agencies and organizations around synergistic research, training, and dissemination and implementation opportunities. With the CDC, it partners on surveillance to guide its early translation research. It has partnered with PCORI to improve the patient-centeredness of research in areas such as blood pressure control and stroke. NIH has also partnered with AHRQ on guidelines development that ties in with its educational mission.

PATIENT-CENTERED OUTCOMES RESEARCH INSTITUTE (PCORI)

"PCORI shares many priorities with AHRQ and NIH, but it comes at these priorities from a different direction," said Joe Selby, PCORI's executive director. The institute's founding legislation directs it to address the questions of stakeholders, including patients, caregivers, clinicians, and payers and purchasers. It does mostly comparative effectiveness research (CER), and this research is primarily conducted through contracts rather than grants, underscoring PCORI's applied

---

4   More information about the center is available at https://ncats.nih.gov/translation/spectrum.

mission and allowing the agency to work closely with its awardees. PCORI is also focused on real-world organizational challenges related to health care.

As with the other agencies described at the workshop, PCORI works collaboratively with a variety of partners, including CDC, the Food and Drug Administration (FDA), and Institutes and Centers of NIH. To date PCORI has worked with AHRQ to navigate its interest in supporting evidence synthesis, dissemination, and workforce training because these three areas have been ones in which AHRQ has historically made investments. This is also true for PCORI's work to understand and assess prevention, diagnosis, and treatment options; to improve health care systems with a particular focus on making care more patient-centered; to eliminate disparities in health care delivery and outcomes; and to promote greater efficiency and transparency in research.

A particular challenge for PCORI is to focus its efforts on the right questions, said Selby. "We work extensively and over prolonged periods with stakeholders to try to get the research questions right." It does less work on comparing new drugs and technologies because "comparative effectiveness research takes time," Selby observed, and such research is difficult to do when products are evolving rapidly, highlighting the need to develop the infrastructure and culture of continuous learning throughout the care process. PCORI also faces the challenge of "who's going to pay for a brand-new technology if insurers have not decided to cover it yet." Finally, it is seeking to establish closer relationships with FDA and CMS to ensure that it can identify the important questions as early in the process as possible.

CENTERS FOR MEDICARE AND MEDICAID SERVICES (CMS)

The Centers for Medicare and Medicaid Services (CMS), the world's largest health insurer, is also a heterogeneous agency with multiple authorities, explained Shari Ling, deputy chief medical officer in the Center for Clinical Standards and Quality at CMS. Its primary mission is not research, but it contributes a small portion of its budget toward evaluating programs and policies. In that respect, its mission coincides with that of health services research.

Central questions for CMS are what services and treatments should be covered, for which populations are they known to be effective as well as safe, and what quality expectations should be met by facilities that participate in Medicare. CMS is aided in its work by AHRQ-supported technology assessments and evidence reviews. Quality expectations can take the form of measures predicated on the evidence that is available, though in some cases evidence is insufficient. In other cases, the research needed to develop measures is insufficient.

CMS has an "incredible opportunity to be an implementation vehicle to help share and spread best practices," said Ling. However, in its work with other entities, it needs to focus very clearly on outcomes that matter. "In general, it's about how do we deliver and pay for care that is of high value."

This observation leads to four challenges. The first is the need for evidence that is applicable to the Medicare population, which is complex and needs programs and policies tailored to its unique needs. The second is the need for data on meaningful outcomes, including not just administrative data but patient-reported outcomes data. The third is the need to see the big picture while running programs and implementing policies that have different origins and multiple goals. The fourth is the need to be mindful of the end users of the research, the programs, and the policies—clinicians at the point of care. According to Ling, CMS needs to ask clinicians, "What do you need that will make your job more effective and easier to translate this body of evidence into outcomes that matter for patients?"

DEPARTMENT OF VETERANS AFFAIRS (VA)

Carolyn Clancy, Deputy Under Secretary for Discovery and Advancement at the Veterans Health Administration, and David Atkins, director of the Health Services Research and Development (HSR&D) Service, both spoke about issues facing the Department of Veterans Affairs (VA).

Many changes have been occurring in the system, noted Atkins. Suicide and posttraumatic stress disorder are now among the VA's top priorities, with more than 50 percent of its patient population having mental health conditions. The VA has been increasing the use of health information technology and telehealth to serve a veteran population that is increasingly rural. It has moved toward patient-centered medical homes, is delivering more care outside VA hospitals, has a long-standing interest in equity and access to care, and is always susceptible to changes caused by changing leadership or priorities. A related issue, Clancy noted, is that the overall nature of health care is changing, which will inevitably affect veterans' health. "We don't even know what a hospital is or is going to be," she noted. Innovations such as micro-hospitals with six to eight beds and extensive digital support could transform the industry.

Building on these themes, Clancy commented that, in her current position, organizational issues are the "top 1-through-10 issues" that she deals with. High reliability can be a fairly abstract topic, but it is essential for the people in VA facilities. These facilities are also subject to hundreds of policies and directives. "It starts to feel a bit like the tyranny of performance measurement," she said.

"We are great at articulating what ought to happen. It is far, far harder to figure out what is happening at any given day in a way that doesn't produce, at least metaphorically, the equivalent of a bureaucrat following every single person around as they do their work." Systems approaches that move beyond measuring single outcomes are one way out of this bind, she said.

In addition, genomics has become a major VA issue. More than 600,000 veterans are now enrolled in the Million Veteran Program, which is "phenomenal," said Clancy.[5] But the genomic information collected as part of the project is not clinically certified, which is one reason why clinicians are not sure how to use it.

The reliability and effectiveness of electronic health records is another issue. The electronic health record does not do anything to people directly, but it can create what she called "perfect storms" in which patient expectations are not met. These expectations also differ among age groups, with many older veterans happy to visit with their friends in waiting rooms, while millennials want an application that lets them know a doctor is running late for an appointment.

The HSR&D program has a dedicated budget of about $100 million and is connected to the integrated health care system of the VA, noted Atkins. It takes advantage of more than two decades of EHR experience and data within the VA, a large number of clinician-investigators, and an obvious audience for its research findings.

However, the research branch of the VA "cannot do it all by ourselves," said Atkins, "so we rely on our other federal partners to share the burden." In recent years, HSR&D has been working with clinical partners to develop research questions to ensure that the answers produced from research are useful to those organizations. In addition, VA research has a broad focus that is driven more by long-term issues than the needs of the moment, despite the fact that the system is often under the microscope and the timeline of policymakers is often not aligned with the timeline of research.

Atkins identified two major opportunities. The first is to work with other organizations on the big problems in health services research that answer fundamental questions. "Those are things that we probably can't fund on our own," he said. The second is to develop ways of sharing information from more limited studies that are useful in addressing broader questions. For example, VA has been developing evaluations of new programs as they are rolled out to answer more basic questions about the design of those programs.

---

5   More information about the program is available at https://www.research.va.gov/mvp.

INTERACTIONS AMONG AGENCIES

The moderator of the session on the health research ecosystem—Atul Grover, executive vice president at the Association of American Medical Colleges—asked individuals from the agencies represented at the session to comment on what they found of value in a specific partnership with another agency.

Atkins mentioned the valuable partnership the VA has forged with the National Center for Complementary and Integrative Health in a pain management collaboratory on the use of nonopioid strategies for combating pain, such as acupuncture, yoga, and massage. Together, the two agencies are funding 11 pragmatic trials that are larger than the VA would be able to fund on its own. "It's a good model of how we can collaborate and bring the advantages of an integrated system [together with] scientific expertise."

Ling noted that, by statute, CMS has to follow the guidelines developed by the US Preventive Services Task Force, "so without the work of AHRQ, we would not be able to implement some of the effective and important preventive interventions." CMS is also working with a variety of agencies, including AHRQ, CDC, VA, and DOD, on reducing events of patient harm. "Those are just a couple of examples of the synergy achieved where CMS actions build on partnerships with others," she said.

Selby pointed to partnerships between PCORI and NIH on pragmatic clinical trials aimed at gathering effectiveness data. PCORI brings a novel perspective to engaging systems and patients within systems, since recruitment remains a challenge. He also mentioned partnerships with AHRQ on dissemination, particularly the dissemination of interventions directed at systems. Mensah cited a partnership with AHRQ on evidence reviews that can be used by professional organizations to develop guidelines in such areas as blood pressure, cholesterol, asthma, and sickle-cell disease. "We don't have the skill set to do that," Mensah said. Khanna mentioned the synergy AHRQ has been able to develop with many of the other agencies represented on the panel. "As they position themselves to serve their customers and users in the future, the question is how AHRQ can help them going forward."

The panelists also briefly discussed their interactions with other agencies not represented at the workshop, such as the Departments of Housing and Urban Development, Transportation, and Labor, which have an important impact on social determinants of health. Such interactions among agencies are rare in Washington, DC, said Atkins, partly because of the way funding oversight is structured in Congress. They typically require "engagement at the highest level, including among the secretaries and in the executive office of the president." When such partnerships do happen, they can be powerful, he added, citing an initiative between the VA and the Department of Housing and Urban Development to reduce homelessness among veterans.

Following up on a suggestion from the audience, the panel briefly discussed the prospects of doing pilot studies and scaling up based on the outcomes of an intervention, whether as part of a collaboration or on their own. Phased research studies are one way to try out innovative ideas, they noted. Some will fail, but others will demonstrate enough promise to progress to larger studies. Such plans can be difficult to get through a review committee, some of the panelists added, but investments in small-scale innovative studies can lead to big returns.

In that regard, Selby asked whether peer review is the best way to get projects of this type evaluated and funded. Research sometimes needs to move faster and more flexibly, resulting in rapid cycles of knowledge production, more robust stakeholder engagement, and the use of indirect costs to build infrastructure for this type of work. He also noted that the health care delivery system is decentralized, which means that many things will continue to happen in silos. "Which organizations are responsible for bringing these silos together?" he asked. "Researchers, funders, payers?"

Mensah noted that the workshop is an opportunity for the leaders in the field to articulate where the field ought to be going. "How much of NIH funding for health services research is enough, and how much is too little? . . . We are limited to some extent, and I'm hoping that you can be as forceful as you can as to how to turn discovery into health impact both at the individual but also at the population level."

3

IMPACT OF HEALTH SERVICES RESEARCH

A session on the impact of health services research on policy and practice revealed a wide range of ways in which knowledge generated by the field has affected health care. It also highlighted the potential role and value of health services research in different contexts and for different audiences, sparking an important discussion of the ways in which the field can serve both policy and practice in the future and laying the groundwork for examination of this topic later in the workshop.

POLICY IMPACT OF HEALTH SERVICES RESEARCH

Health services research is as complicated as the health system that it tries to elucidate, said David Blumenthal, president and chief executive officer of the Commonwealth Fund. As a result, translating its results into terms that are useful to policy makers can be difficult. Nevertheless, health services research has made important contributions to policy in such areas as cost sharing, quality, payment models, and patient safety, Blumenthal observed. In particular, he identified 10 studies that have influenced policy (Box 3-1) and briefly described several of them.

In their discussion of how rates of utilization varied from town to town and county to county in Vermont, Wennberg and Gittelsohn (1973) raised the issue of practice variation that continues to be studied and have implications for the public and private sectors today.

McGlynn et al. (2003) showed that only about 55 percent of encounters with physicians resulted in the receipt of recommended care and has been an important influence on work on health care quality ever since.

Brook et al. (2006) described the RAND Health Insurance Experiment, which was "probably the largest and most influential single randomized control trial that has ever been done—and may ever be done—in health services research," said Blumenthal. It documented the effects of cost sharing on the consumption

BOX 3–1
Ten Influential Studies in Health Services Research

1. Wennberg, J., and A. Gittelsohn. 1973. Small area variations in health care delivery: a population-based health information system can guide planning and regulatory decision-making. *Science* 182(4117):1102-1108.
2. Starfield, B., J. Weiner, L. Mumford, and D. Steinwachs. 1991. Ambulatory care groups: a categorization of diagnoses for research and management. *Health Services Research* 26(1):53-74.
3. McGlynn, E. A., S. M. Asch, J. Adams, J. Keesey, K. Hicks, A. DeCristofaro, and E. A. Kerr, 2003. The quality of health care delivered to adults in the United States. *New England Journal of Medicine* 348(26):2635-2645.
4. Brook, R. H., E. B. Keeler, K. N. Lohr, J. P. Newhouse, J. E. Ware, W. H. Rogers, A. R. Davies, C. D. Sherbourne, G. A. Goldberg, P. Camp, C. Kamberg, A. Leibowitz, J. Keesey, and D. Reboussin, 2006. The health insurance experiment: a classic RAND study speaks to the current health care reform debate. Santa Monica, CA: RAND Corporation.
5. Campbell, E. G., J. S. Weissman, S. Ehringhaus, S. R. Rao, B. Moy, S. Feibelmann, and S. D. Goold. 2007. Institutional academic-industry relationships. *JAMA* 298(15):1779-1786.
6. Girosi, F., A. Cordova, C. Eibner, C. R. Gresenz, E. B. Keeler, J. S. Ringel, J. Sullivan, J. Bertko, M. B. Buntin, and R. Vardavas. 2009. Overview of the COMPARE microsimulation model. Santa Monica, CA: RAND Corporation.
7. Baiker, K., S. L. Taubman, H. L. Allen, M. Bernstein, J. H. Gruber, J. P. Newhouse, E. C. Schneider, B. J. Wright, A. M. Zaslavsky, and A. N. Finkelstein; Oregon Health Study Group. 2013. The Oregon experiment—effects of Medicaid on clinical outcomes. *New England Journal of Medicine* 368(18):1713-1722.
8. Lee, J. L., M. Maciejewski, S. Raju, W. H. Shrank, and N. K. Choudhry. 2013. Value-based insurance design: quality improvement but no cost savings. *Health Affairs* 32(7):1251-1257.
9. Song, Z., S. Rose, D. G. Safran, B. E. Landon, M. P. Day, and M. E. Chernew. 2014. Changes in health care spending and quality 4 years into global payment. *New England Journal of Medicine* 371(18):1704-1714.
10. Sommers, B. D., B. Maylone, R. J. Blendon, E. J. Orav, and A. M. Epstein. 2017. Three-year impacts of the affordable care act: improved medical care and health among low-income adults. *Health Affairs* 36(6):1119-1128.

SOURCE: David Blumenthal. Presentation to the National Academy of Medicine, February 2018.

of care, on the use of appropriate and inappropriate services (showing that cost sharing reduces the use of services but does not reduce the use of inappropriate services), and on health. The result has been an important conversation that helped inform the creation of the Patient Protection and Affordable Care Act.

Campbell et al. (2007), in a project with which Blumenthal was involved, looked at interactions between academia and industry and contributed to passage of the Sunshine Act part of the Patient Protection and Affordable Care Act, which made it possible to learn if a physician is accepting donations or gifts from the pharmaceutical industry.

Girosi et al. (2009) developed one of only a very limited number of microsimulation models for health care available to predict the effects of new policies. Of the others, one has been developed by the Urban Institute, and another, developed by the Congressional Budget Office, is not available to health services researchers.

Song et al. (2014) evaluated the alternative quality contract, which was important in informing the accountable care organization model and demonstrated the potential to save money and improve quality by providing global budgets to physician groups.

Sommers et al. (2017) documented that expansion of Medicaid improved the health and well-being of low-income populations compared with states that did not expand Medicaid, a finding relevant to recent discussions of block granting for Medicaid.

Many more studies could be listed, Blumenthal said, but these 10 are enough to demonstrate "that this work deeply affects policy and also deeply affects the way the health system operates."

QUALITY AND SAFETY IMPACT OF HEALTH SERVICES RESEARCH

As a specific example of the impacts of health services research, the president and chief executive officer of the Leapfrog Group, Leah Binder, noted that her organization, which represents employers and other purchasers of health benefits, relies heavily on health services research. "It gives us the insights we need to understand where the problem is, what are the best methods for solving it, and how to hold people accountable for results."

Binder focused first on the problem of detecting and preventing mistakes. Health services research has provided key tools to identify errors, provide insights into how they happen, and determine how they can be prevented. Hospitals can now be held more accountable both internally, in terms of physicians and clinicians holding each other accountable for results, and externally, through businesses and other purchasers of health care gaining more accountability. "We can look at results across the board and compare among health systems to better understand who is reaching and achieving at the highest levels and who is not and who needs to work on it." This is information that would have been impossible to envision in the 1980s, yet now is available routinely because of health services research.

Binder also cited the progress that has been made through the development of patient safety indicators. "There's been a lot of criticism of them, but they are extraordinarily effective." Patient safety indicators have been endorsed by the National Quality Forum, extensively validated and tested, and utilized in research and in efforts to improve accountability. "We rely heavily on them, and we've seen hospital systems embrace them and make real changes that have been very effective in saving lives."

She highlighted the annual survey that Leapfrog conducts, in which about half of US hospitals voluntarily make data available on patient care. As an example of the survey's value, it includes data on the results of a Computerized Provider Order Entry (CPOE) assessment, which was developed with funding from AHRQ, that evaluates a hospital's CPOE system. Provided with a set of dummy patients and dummy orders, the hospital determines if the system alerts to common errors embedded in the orders. "Most hospitals, when they take this test for the first time, are shocked because they thought their system was working just fine, and they usually find out it's not," said Binder. Based on her experience, about a third of the orders that they tested each year—and about one in six orders that would result in fatalities—were not alerted. But when hospitals take the test for a second time, they generally improve. "To me, [that] has been an example of where excellent health services research can make a difference both in quality improvement and accountability and has saved lives."

Looking toward the future, Binder suggested that people think of measures and measurement not just as a noun, but as a verb. Sometimes, instead of a new measure, new strategies to achieve measurement are needed, she said. For example, the use of social media makes it possible to interact with consumers in ways that can improve their health. This work is in its infancy, she noted, but already other industries provide models that could be adopted in health care. In addition, she lauded the requirement by PCORI to incorporate patient views into the research it funds.

Binder concluded by warning that the battles over the status of AHRQ could be discouraging the next generation of researchers from entering the field. This "would be a terrible tragedy," she said, "because so many of the problems in our health care system can be solved only through excellence in health services research."

HEALTH SERVICES RESEARCH
IN A LARGE HEALTH CARE SYSTEM

Following passage of the Patient Protection and Affordable Care Act, Partners Healthcare founded a large accountable care organization to manage risk-based reimbursement models. On January 1, 2012, Partners transitioned from having financial risk for the costs of its 100,000 employees and dependents to having financial risk for the cost of an additional 350,000 commercially insured patients and 100,000 Medicare patients. Then, on March 1, 2018, the at-risk population expanded to more than 85 percent of all patients seen in primary care, because the system agreed to accept financial risk for the cost of care for all its Medicaid patients. "If you haven't heard about what's going on in Massachusetts, it's a landmark event," said Timothy Ferris, a practicing primary care physician and chief executive officer of Massachusetts General Physicians Organization.

As senior vice president for population health at Partners Healthcare, Ferris was faced with the task of replacing the delivery of existing services with services that produce higher value across the full spectrum of health care services. Informed by health services research, the framework developed to meet this task had three main components.

The first was a change management task focused on motivating the 65,000 people working in the Partners Healthcare system to change the care they deliver. Health services research "knocked it out of the park" on that part of the framework, he said. The definitive literature on gaps in quality, quality metrics, risk adjustment, practice variation, experience of care, and on safety and errors have been critically important to accomplishing this task. He added one caveat, which is that the extrapolation of studies with wide error bars from a single site or a handful of sites to a national estimate, while perhaps helpful in a political process, can be destructive in trying to make changes within an organization. "Exaggerating the problem can be counterproductive to a change process."

The second component was to define service delivery changes that presented the greatest opportunities for improvement. In this case, Ferris said health services research was "helpful, but it could have been more helpful." Mongan et al. (2008) listed the topic areas involved in slowing the growth of health care costs: payment reform effectiveness review for new technology, electronic health record (EHR) research, care coordination for complex illness, transparency, reduction in administrative costs, drug pricing reform, and enhanced prevention. "I would give the history of health services research on these topics a solid B, maybe a B plus," Ferris said. He also said that two other areas should be added to the list. The first is variation research using claims data and clinical data, which can produce very different results. The second is artificial intelligence, which enhances our ability to analyze data and perform complex analytic tasks.

For this task, he also listed a caveat: from a manager's perspective, research is often either too general or too specific in identifying opportunities to improve care. Economists have a tendency to draw "sweeping conclusions from oversimplified models of care delivery using data generated for a different purpose." At the same time, health services research can be full of clinical detail but lack relevance. Ferris said that he has tried to occupy a space between these two worlds and recommended the paper by Eisenberg et al. (2000) on transforming insurance coverage into quality medical care as "the best articulation of how to think about the problem faced by managers who need to improve service delivery."

The third component was to design, build, test, and disseminate interventions that clearly demonstrate improved value. In this case, he said, health services research has been "occasionally helpful, sometimes counterproductive, and mostly irrelevant." The problem boils down to the difference between efficacy and effectiveness research. Programs and practices can be implemented in many different ways, since there are many different solutions to an operational problem. Doing randomized trials of actual changes in care delivery involve such artificial conditions as patient consent, a stable exposure, and relatively short durations, all of which provide a distorted sense of what happens in real life to such an extent that the results of such trials, especially when they are negative, are largely irrelevant, he stated. "Time and again, we have implemented changes in care delivery where there is existing research that says it cannot be done, and yet we have found success. . . . There's a wide gap between the statement that a particular trial did not work, indicating that the specifics of the trial should be used to learn how not to do something, and saying that the idea behind the trial is itself not possible to achieve. This seems obvious, but like all researchers, health services researchers can push the limits of the generalizability of their results." At the same time, and "on a more positive note," he pointed to an extremely important negative trial—the Study to Understand Prognoses and Preferences for Outcomes and Risks of Treatments (SUPPORT) trial funded by RWJF (The SUPPORT Principal Investigators, 1995). "That negative trial has very heavily influenced what we have done to improve end-of-life care."

He concluded by pointing out how important health services researchers have been to change efforts at Partners Healthcare. "Time after time, our team is asked by various internal stakeholders to justify our expenditures, our focus, our approach. Having a small team of skilled health services researchers has been essential to our efforts and has led to countless presentations important for sustaining momentum within our organization and more than 60 publications in the past six years to try to disseminate our largely observational trials."

APPLYING HEALTH SERVICES RESEARCH IN PRACTICE AND POLICY

The presenters' examination of past advances in health services research led to a discussion of the many ways in which the field could affect policy and practice in the future. As Blumenthal pointed out, health services research can address everything from large health systems reforms and policy issues using traditional research methods to specific implementation issues that apply in particular contexts. With regard to the former set of problems, health services research can be extremely useful in identifying the most pressing health and cost problems and also possibly in designing macro-level policies. When he was working on implementing EHRs, he was guided by the conviction that having such data available would create huge benefits—and now advances such as those in artificial intelligence are proving that conviction correct. But this conviction required "an understanding of the interaction between data and progress in a field that is informed by research."

Health services research has been less impactful on micro-level implementation decisions, he continued. One reason is that such problems tend to be less suited to traditional academic research approaches. Those who study such problems therefore may need to be rewarded in other ways than through the traditional academic award structure. For example, he pointed out that health services research has rarely supported or guided in a definitive way the decisions he has had to make as a health system manager. The difficulty has been both finding literature that is relevant and applying that literature if and when it is found. For that reason, he has always encouraged the researchers who have worked with him to experiment in the practical world and spend time as implementers or government officials if they can, "because it leads to a completely different set of questions rising to the surface." He also encouraged researchers to ensure that their work is driven by practical purposes and that the applicability of their results is appropriately described.

He acknowledged, however, that this advice ignores some of the tenets of academic training and the culture of research, where new researchers are told to pick a single area and dig as deeply as they can into that topic. Young researchers may also be discouraged from working in government, serving as a manager, or even doing translational research because they will fall off the promotion track. Such advice represents an "endemic academic debility that health services research has to contend with," he said. "Being grounded in academics is both a great strength and also a great limitation."

Alan Weil, the editor-in-chief of *Health Affairs*, called attention to the importance of translating results from health services research, commenting that translation of research involves a different skill set than academic research and is not primarily about publishing papers. "Diffusion [of knowledge] is a more complex and multifactorial process than publishing journal papers," he said. "If we want to maximize value, we need to think about it in the context of diffusion, not just about the creation of health services research."

Similarly, Ferris also drew a distinction between academic health services research geared toward academic purposes and research geared toward implementation questions. The differences between these types of research have implications for training, hiring, and the dissemination of knowledge that have not always been well recognized, he noted. For example, implementation science can aggregate methods from health services research and business and management science while also using new analytic approaches.

He emphasized that the central issue is the dissemination of useful information, not just the publication of papers or the pursuit of high-impact factor journals. As an example of such research, he pointed to the publications he and his colleagues are producing, which typically are observational studies of problems and of how changes affected those problems one way or the other. However, such studies "do not make the grade for evidence in the way we traditionally think of evidence," he noted, and they are difficult to publish in prominent journals.

Binder pointed out that health services research cannot and should not attempt to answer all the questions a leader in a health system might have about how to improve, given the difficulties of running a health system. But when leaders are motivated to make changes, they typically are able to do so, even if those changes can only be guided and not dictated by research. "There's a certain magic to leadership and culture and management that remains yours, but research can inform that." Research can also compare one system to another, which can help systems understand where they need to go. It can suggest ways of incentivizing improvement while leaving the challenge of change management to health system leaders.

At the same time, Binder pointed to the fundamental value of health services research in providing ways of thinking about value and cost effectiveness in specific and actionable ways. For example, "if there's any consensus in our health care system, it's that we have to move away from fee-for-service. We just haven't been able to figure out how to do it, and there are lots of reasons for that. But no field has given us more tools to do that than health services research." As a specific example, she cited the track record of health services research in developing concepts and methods that enable comparisons among providers and health systems, which has been "an extraordinary accomplishment."

4

GUIDING HEALTH SYSTEM PERFORMANCE IMPROVEMENT

New tools and approaches in health services research are poised to contribute major advances in care quality and efficiency. Developments in predictive analytics and artificial intelligence, models and agreements for large database sharing and analysis, care culture and shared decision-making instruments, and economic and incentive modeling approaches are all examples of advancing health services research capacities. In addition, factors such as how health systems are organized, led, and reformed can improve the care that is delivered, ultimately leading to better outcomes for health care consumers.

PREDICTIVE ANALYTICS AND ARTIFICIAL INTELLIGENCE

Rainu Kaushal, chair and Nanette Laitman Distinguished Professor of Healthcare Policy and Research at Weill Cornell Medicine and chief of healthcare research and policy at the New York-Presbyterian Hospital/Weill Cornell Medical Center, focused on predictive modeling and artificial intelligence, which she described as having "tremendous promise as we start to look forward in health care delivery and in health services research."

With funding from PCORI, Kaushal and her team have been looking at the 10 percent of high-need, high-cost patients who account for 50 percent of health care costs. Taking advantage of rich clinical, claims, and social determinants data, and incorporating literature reviews and perspectives from patients, clinicians, and health systems leaders, these investigators developed a taxonomy of computable phenotypes to characterize high-need, high-cost patients in order to help target effective interventions. Using data from PCORnet and from Medicare, they were able to link 1 million Medicare beneficiaries with clinical data, and they had nine-digit ZIP codes for 225,000 patients. "That becomes important, because that's how we began to understand the social determinant piece," Kaushal said. Despite the bluntness of ZIP codes as a measure of social determinants, "we were still able to elicit some very meaningful information."

The team ultimately identified ten medical and behavioral computable phenotypes and calculated the percentage of high-need, high-cost patients within each category. In particular, using the data described above, the team identified a social vulnerability index that described high-need, high-cost patients.

In response to these efforts, three health systems have already pledged funding to translate these computable phenotypes into actionable algorithms using the types of data that the health systems have in hand. Collaborators at the Anthem insurance company are also seeking to translate the data into meaningful variables for the commercially insured. Additional work has focused and will focus on the availability of structured, linkable data, Logical Observation Identifiers Names and Codes (LOINC) laboratory data and the matching of payment and care delivery models to categories of patients.

Kaushal emphasized three principles derived from this work. The first is the importance of multiple sources of data and the ability to link those to social determinants data. The second is that health services research needs to be actionable, whether in terms of new health care delivery models or policy. The third is the importance of patient and stakeholder engagement. "Having patients and stakeholders not only providing input but also actually solving problems together in the same room is what makes the work we do so much richer and so much more meaningful."

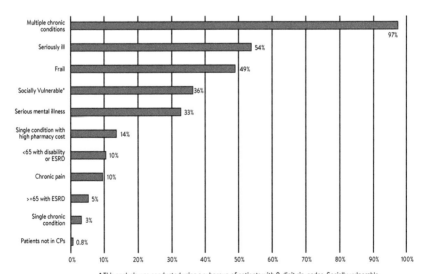

* This analysis was conducted using a subgroup of patients with 9-digit zip-codes. Socially vulnerable patients were defined as individuals whose social index is in the top 30%.

FIGURE 1-1 The percentage of high-need, high-cost patients by computable phenotype.

SOURCE: Rainu Kaushal. Presentation to the National Academy of Medicine. February 2018.

IDENTIFYING APPROACHES TO PAYING
FOR POPULATION HEALTH

Building on the theme of action-oriented efforts, Dana Safran, chief performance measurement and improvement officer and senior vice president of enterprise analytics at Blue Cross Blue Shield of Massachusetts, described the effort within Blue Cross Blue Shield of Massachusetts to develop a new contract model that would improve quality and outcomes while significantly slowing the rate of growth in health care spending. The result was an approach called the Alternative Quality Contract (AQC). "The uptake of the model happened quite quickly," said Safran. The model is based on long-term, generally five-year, contracts that establish sustained partnerships and support ongoing investments and commitments to improvement. The contracts specify a global budget for a population, covering the full continuum of care and adjusted by health status. They also employ a set of quality and outcome measures to motivate the improvement of care. The intention is to avoid both overuse and underuse, said Safran. "The quality measures have served a very important role in terms of avoiding the stunting of care that we might fear would happen when you go to a budget model." Echoing a point made earlier by Leah Binder (see chapter 3), Safran observed that developing these quality measures would have been impossible without health services research.

The AQC was evaluated from its first year (Song et al. 2014). After four years, it had clearly bent the cost curve—"interestingly, more and more each year," said Safran. Furthermore, it significantly improved quality and outcomes and helped close long-standing health disparities (Song et al. 2017). These disparities were closed even though the AQC does not adjust quality measures by socioeconomic status (SES). "I couldn't bring myself to say we're going to set a lower bar in our performance measure for organizations that serve lower SES populations, so we set the same bar for everybody. What happened in our network was pretty remarkable, because organizations that serve the lowest socioeconomic groups were some of the ones that rose from the very lowest levels of performance to surpassing many of the organizations that served a higher SES mix," said Safran.

One place where health services research has not come into play is in studying how organizations have adapted their delivery system model to achieve the results the AQC has had, Safran pointed out. Still, the absence of that research has not stopped organizations from being creative, testing new methods, learning from others and from best practice-sharing forums, and using the literature to improve quality and cost.

Safran pointed to four domains in which AQC groups have been innovating while reducing overall spending: staffing models, approaches to patient engagement, data systems and health information technology, and referral relationships and integration across settings. She particularly highlighted patient-reported outcomes as "measures that tell us whether what we are doing in health care is working, whether people are feeling better and functioning better because of what we're doing." Of the five high-prevalence, high-cost conditions where few quality and outcome measures exist—cardiovascular, orthopedics, oncology, mental health, and obstetrics—Blue Cross Blue Shield of Massachusetts began by introducing patient-reported outcome measures in two areas: depression and hip and knee pain. In 2016, these measures were extended to lower-back pain, prostate cancer, all cancer with active treatment, and coronary-artery disease. The data from these measures can be used to predict who will benefit from certain procedures. Some patients are likely to benefit from a hip or knee replacement, others are likely not to benefit, and for patients in the middle, other factors can impact the care management decision. "Imagine having data like that for shared decision making with our patients in other areas," Safran concluded. Such information will clearly "get some of the wasteful care out of our delivery system."

ENGINEERING HEALTH SYSTEM TRANSFORMATION

Bolstered by health services research findings on the results from the application of engineering principles in health care, more and more health care organizations are implementing systems engineering innovations. As an example of successful health systems engineering, Gary Kaplan, chairman and chief executive officer of the Virginia Mason Health System, described the system's deployment of the Toyota production system to health care. Eighteen years ago, when the process started, Virginia Mason stated that its customer was the patient. But the board "wouldn't let us accept that," said Kaplan. "They said, 'If that's the case, why do things look the way they do?'" A deep dive into the system then revealed that care was organized around the needs of doctors, nurses, pharmacists, and others working in the system. "The example I always use are waiting rooms, where we spend millions of dollars in this country every year to build spaces so that patients can hurry up to be on time and wait for us. It is the antithesis of patient-centered care."

The result has been a sustained effort to achieve large-scale culture change through the conscious deployment of a new management system. Virginia Mason found that system not in other health care systems but in the Boeing Corporation. Boeing was using the Toyota production system, which Virginia Mason soon embraced as not just a process improvement method but as "the way we run the entire organization."

Kaplan explained that Virginia Mason views quality as a function of delivering appropriate care, improving outcomes, providing high-quality service, and reducing waste. Also critical is ensuring deep respect for individuals within the system through actions such as expressing gratitude and being a team player.

In implementing the Toyota production system, Virginia Mason has seized on an approach known as "experience-based design," which Kaplan defined as a philosophy and set of methods focused on understanding the experiences and emotions of those who are involved in delivering and receiving health care. For example, it has generated a list of words that are either positive, neutral, or negative and has made them part of the system's improvement methods, which has enabled it to measure improvements in patient and team member emotional responses.

Among the variables necessary to transform an organization, Kaplan cited a sense of urgency, visible and committed leadership, a shared vision, and aligned expectations. In addition, the current environment requires a continued acceleration of improvement results, he said, given the increased pace of change, the need for increased quality outcomes and reduced costs, and the threat of stress and burnout. Documenting these improvements requires a focus on measurement, which Virginia Mason has achieved by working with other organizations.

Virginia Mason is now in version 2.0 of its production system, which incorporates respect for people and continuous improvement to enhance the flow of health care. At this point, organizations from Japan and other countries are sending teams to the medical center to learn how to apply the Toyota methods, said Kaplan. He concluded by quoting the philosopher Eric Hoffer: "In times of change, learners inherit the earth, while the learned find themselves beautifully equipped to deal with the world that no longer exists."

Speaking to the challenges faced by organizations seeking to make culture changes of the magnitude required, Kevin Schulman, now professor of medicine at Stanford University, pointed out that a business model is a fixed characteristic of an organization that is resilient and resistant to incremental change. Organizations are designed to produce predictable results, and they do that by building stable cultures. Changes in an organization's leadership do not automatically make a difference, because people in the organization know the culture and how to behave. This observation applies as much to medical centers as to other organizations, Schulman said. When leaders ask organizations to make changes, "it's going to be a long time before you get the kind of performance changes you want."

One way to spur innovation in an organization is to name a chief innovation officer, Schulman observed. But when one of his students surveyed 25 chief innovation officers at large health systems in the United States, she found that the median budgets of the offices of the Chief Innovation Officer were $3.5 million, in organizations with annual budgets that can measure in the billions of dollars (Shah et al, 2018). "The marketing budget when you do a name change is [typically] bigger than the chief innovation officer budgets," Schulman observed.

In recent years, the greatest changes in the values of goods and services have come from the high-tech side of the economy. Health care, meanwhile, has struggled to bend the cost curve. "That's our challenge," Schulman said. "What kind of innovation do we want? How does health services research help us describe the innovation that is needed?" Innovation, according to Schulman, is likely to come from nimble and flexible organizations. "That's where we're going to see the huge value creation in the economy." As one example of where innovation could make a difference, he pointed out that billing for primary care services accounts for 14.5 percent of the total cost, and billing for emergency services takes 25 percent (Tseng et al. 2018). "There are plenty of places where we could see huge innovations," and where engineering principles can foster improvement.

PROMOTING AND MEASURING CULTURE CHANGE

The panel was challenged by the moderator, Jay Want, executive director of the Peterson Center on Healthcare, to say whether it was possible to identify high-value systems, given the importance of culture in those systems and the difficulty of measuring it. Schulman pointed out that culture builds up over a long period of time and that it is difficult to measure culture objectively. It is also difficult, he added, to measure the impact of leaders on an organization's culture.

Kaplan argued that health services research needs to develop ways of measuring culture, though Virginia Mason has made progress on measuring subcultures to link staff engagement, patient satisfaction, and a culture of safety to strong managers or weak managers. But measures of end-user value are also important, he said. "The evidence-based process measures that are clearly associated with superior outcomes need to continue to be measured." To this, Kaushal added that it is critical to use clinical, rather than claims, data for outcome measurement, which will become increasingly possible with the increased structuring of clinical data and more advanced natural language processing.

In response to a question, Kaplan pointed out that the changes instituted in his system have not been based on research, because not much research is available on such changes, particularly as they relate to institutional culture. "When you are the first to go forward, you're kind of flying blind." But these and similar experiences could lend themselves to research on the impact of culture, he added. However, Charles (Chip) Kahn, of the Federation of American Hospitals (FAH), made the additional point that most hospital organizations have relatively small market shares, which makes widespread cultural change more difficult. The centrality of culture to sustained organizational success, in combination with the underdeveloped state of the science base on factors that shape culture change, is testament to its importance as a health services research focus.

MEASURING VALUE

Similarly, Safran pointed out that measuring value is difficult, especially since most current measures have grown out of a fee-for-service era. By measuring results, it is possible to link value-based payments to outcome-oriented measure sets. "If we systematically incorporated patient-reported outcome measures into all of the clinical areas [to show] a measurable change in how somebody is feeling or functioning, then we could tell you who to invest that capital in and who not to, but we don't have that today. We have just a few outcome measures on things that you know are important, but they're not everything, and they're certainly not what's important to patients."

Lee Fleischer, from the University of Pennsylvania Perelman School of Medicine, raised the issue of complications in measuring outcomes and understanding value such as the placebo effect, since patients may feel better after having a procedure even though the procedure would not be judged appropriate on other measures. Kaplan acknowledged the "complex interaction between a needy consumer and a willing provider." As an example, he pointed out that, among the patients sent by physicians to Virginia Mason for complex spine surgery, only 1 percent of those subsequently go on to have surgery. "It's not that people have malintent," he said. The problem is the unintended consequences of overuse by both consumers and providers, "and we have to attack both of those."

Mark Pauly, Bendheim Professor in the Department of Health Care Management at The Wharton School and Professor of Economics in the School of Arts and Sciences at the University of Pennsylvania, commented that most businesses do not get tangled up in outcome measures. Their outcomes are whether people are willing to pay money for the goods and services they provide. Health care is different in that people are not used to thinking that way, though they can be encouraged to ask and answer such questions—such as how much money they would be willing to pay for an extra quality-adjusted life year. The health care system also can be structured so that consumers must make choices across health plans affiliated with different systems so that they can consciously think about their tradeoffs. Schulman pointed out that one issue is the disconnect between the amount consumers are willing to pay for insurance and the costs of expensive procedures and treatments, such as treatments for cancer. For this reason, he said, "implementing a low-cost health plan can be impossible."

As health services research is increasingly called upon to define and elaborate on the value proposition under circumstances in which the balances among individuals, societal, and commercial perspectives contribute substantial complexity, it will be all the more important to have systematic, transparent, and multistakeholder public engagement.

5

BRIDGING HEALTH AND SOCIAL SERVICES TO IMPROVE CARE ACCESS

A long-time priority of health services research has been a focus on issues affecting access to care, including community factors, the availability of social services, and the social determinants of health. Social determinants of health have been defined by Healthy People 2020 as "conditions in the environments in which people are born, live, learn, work, play, worship, and age that affect a wide range of health, functioning, and quality-of-life outcomes and risks." These issues, among others, result in a rich network of interlinked issues for health services researchers.

UNDERSTANDING SOCIAL DETERMINANTS OF HEALTH

The social determinants of health are ubiquitous and have a significant impact on health outcomes, said Sandro Galea, dean and Robert A. Knox Professor at Boston University School of Public Health. "You can't avoid thinking about ubiquitous determinants if you want to get insight that informs the kind of questions that health services research is trying to get at."

Health systems are starting to realize the power of this observation. For example, the Boston Medical Center is investing $6.5 million in affordable housing to enhance health in the community, improve patient outcomes, and reduce medical costs. On its website, the CDC has called attention to several such factors that have a direct and measurable effect on health:

- With rehabilitating housing, 62 percent of adults have excellent health versus 33 percent without such housing.
- In a city of a million residents, a 40 percent expansion in transit development has an annual health benefit of $216 million.

- Early childhood education has a benefit-to-cost ratio of 5 to 1 with a reduction in crime rates, child maltreatment, teen pregnancy, and academic problems.
- Each time the Earned Income Tax Credit increases by 10 percent, infant mortality drops by 23.2 per 100,000 population.

Galea is the coauthor, with Katherine Keyes, of the book *Population Health Science*, from which he drew two conclusions that are directly relevant for health services research (Keyes and Galea, 2016). The first is that the magnitude of an effect of exposure on disease is dependent on the prevalence of the factors that interact with that exposure. For example, three studies might look at the effects of an intervention on hypertension, with one finding no effect and the other two finding effects of different sizes. One interpretation is that two of the studies were wrong, but that is "not necessarily the case," said Galea. Rather, the intervention may need to happen along with exposure to other conditions to have an effect. If the intervention and a social condition are both necessary but insufficient causes of an outcome, then the outcome will occur only when both are present. If all, none, or some members of a population are exposed to the social condition, outcomes will vary accordingly when they are exposed to the intervention. The challenge with ubiquitous conditions is that their influence cannot be separated out because they "affect everybody, all of us, all the time," said Galea. Proper inferences in health services research, therefore, need to take these ubiquitous forces into account.

The second principle he cited is that small changes in ubiquitous causes may result in more substantial changes in the health of populations than larger changes in rarer causes. Galea cited the metaphor of goldfish in a fishbowl that are given plenty of food but die because their water is never changed. Another example is early research on babies whose mothers used crack cocaine that found an association between crack cocaine use and developmental delay. However, long-term studies found that the overriding predictor of developmental delay was exposure to extreme poverty and lack of environmental stimulation. "We missed the presence of the ubiquitous factor."

Galea drew three implications from these observations. First, "you simply can't forget ubiquitous causes." Second, researchers need to focus on what matters most. Third, health is not a dichotomous outcome and needs to be considered more broadly as a continuous outcome. "We hinge our inference on stories that are simpler than the reality," he concluded. All research endeavors must therefore focus on the systemic context of issues being studied.

MOVING RESEARCH INTO COMMUNITIES

Building on the themes from Galea's presentation, Jack Westfall, medical director of whole-person care at Santa Clara Valley Medical Center, observed that most of the people in the community are not getting health care in the places where health services researchers get much of their data. In a classic article on the ecology of medical care, White et al. (1961) displayed graphically that of 1,000 people in a community, 750 experience illness or injury in a given month, 250 seek primary care, 10 are hospitalized, and 1 is hospitalized in an academic health center (Figure 5-1). This assessment was repeated in 2000 and in 2016 (Green et al. 2001; Johansen et al. 2016) with similar conclusions.

Not much is known, Westfall pointed out, about the interface between the 10 people who are hospitalized and the 250 people who are seen in an ambulatory setting, or between the people seen in the ambulatory setting and the 500 who experience illness or injury during that month but do not seek care, or between the 750 who experience an illness or injury and the 250 who remain well in a given month.

Innovation moves into the community through the types of research along stages of a translational continuum represented as T1 through T4 in Figure 5-2, connoting the progress from basic research to the implementation of research in the community. T1 and T2 research occurs mostly at academic institutions. Laboratory discoveries are translated into human pathophysiology. New pills, procedures, and devices are translated into treatments and disease-modifying management programs. But new discoveries also must be translated into clinical practice in real-world settings, where patients and communities can provide the context for new discoveries and lead to locally relevant and meaningful programs and language. T3 and T4 research moves findings from academic institutions into the world of integrated primary care and population health, where data to ask and answer questions about translating discovery in a few to the many begin to accrue. These different kinds of research line up with the boxes in the ecology of medical care, Westfall observed. Much of the early research is done in the institution, while much of the practice-based and community research is done in the larger boxes.

These observations are not new, Westfall pointed out. In 1967, Marion Folsom published the book *Health is a Community Affair*, which made the point that education, food security, safe housing, legal services, and other factors all combine to impact individual and community health (Folsom, 1967; Folsom Group, 2012). From this perspective, health care problems occur in the community, not in the smaller boxes of the ecology of health care (Figure 5-2). They encompass public health, community services, and primary care. The judicial system, food deserts, education levels, safe housing, and human services "all conspire to impact health care and health care utilization."

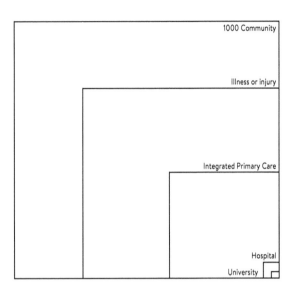

FIGURE 5-1 | "Kerr White" boxes describe the number of people, from each 1,000 in a community, who experience an illness or injury in a month, receive ambulatory care, are hospitalized, and are hospitalized in an academic medical center.
SOURCE: White at al. 1961

Health services research must ensure that it is assessing the ultimate impact of forces on system-wide performance and health outcomes, Westfall observed. It can work at the level of integrated primary care, at the community level, or with people who are experiencing the social determinants of health but are not yet suffering consequences to their health. Traditional academic research increases understanding of what happens when prevention does not occur or illness is not treated. Health services research can define the parameters of prevention, measure the impact and develop interventions for the disintegrated social determinants of health, and ask and answer questions that matter to more people more of the time. "However, we've seen a disproportionate share of health services research time and resources spent on the small boxes in the lower right-hand corner," said Westfall, where hospital claims data and electronic health record data tend to be available. "Health services research has gravitated to where the data are." A primary challenge for the field is shaping the capacity to account for and assess system factors in play.

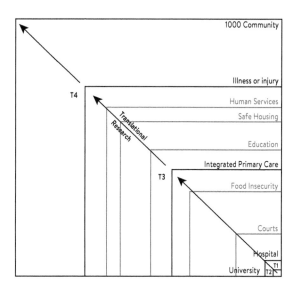

FIGURE 3-2 Translational research can move results derived from hospitalized patients into the community.
SOURCE: Adapted from White et al. 1961

Focusing on the ubiquitous determinants of health in social and community settings can link the small boxes with the much larger boxes. It can also help meet needs in the clinic, community, and broader population. In the exam room, providers need discoveries to work for individual patients given their unique biology, family, neighborhood, values, and choices. In an integrated primary care clinic, providers and their staff need discoveries that they can offer safely with high fidelity and quality. At the community level, they need discoveries that patients will seek out and accept, that are available, and that align with the values of the community. At the population level, they need discoveries that are affordable, that make the world a better place, and that balance the needs of the individual, practice, and community.

EFFECTS OF HEALTH INSURANCE BENEFIT DESIGN

Within the health care system, consumers can be engaged in their care through a variety of mechanisms, including shared decision-making, case management, health navigators, and benefit design. Michael Chernew, Leonard D. Schaeffer Professor of Health Care Policy and director of the Healthcare Markets and Regulation Lab in the Department of Health Care Policy at Harvard Medical School, discussed the last of these options. It is not the only and may not even be the best way to involve consumers in health care decisions, he said, but it has been the focus of much innovative health services research.

Annual health care deductibles have been rising much faster than inflation or earnings since 2011. Deductibles are designed to improve incentives for health care consumers by reducing excess use of health care and encouraging price shopping. However, there are three problems with this approach. Prices for health care are high, some health care services are overused, and some are underused. Patients do respond to cost sharing (Brook et al. 2006). When they are charged more, they use less care. However, "consumers aren't great shoppers," Chernew noted. "They cut back on appropriate use and inappropriate use in the exact same amount." Copays reduce the use of preventive services and beneficial pharmaceuticals (Sui et al. 1986). "It's amazing how little you can charge somebody and have them not take their preventive medicines or use preventive services." The overall picture, said Chernew, quoting a friend, is that "the United States has *Star Wars* medicine and *Flintstone* financing."

"Nuances" can be a critical influence in benefit design, said Chernew. For example, use of a tiered network design can steer patients away from nonpreferred to preferred hospitals (Frank et al. 2015). Benefit designs can affect whether patients choose high-price or low-price hospitals for knee- or hip-replacement surgery (Robinson and Brown, 2013). The structuring of copayments can increase adherence to medications (Chernew, 2008).

The problem with nuances is that they can be complicated, Chernew admitted. "The challenge for health services research going forward is how nuanced can we be" and to identify innovative nuances that decrease spending without negatively impacting outcomes for patients. For example, straightforward price transparency tools are not associated with lower outpatient spending (Desai et al. 2016); instead, patients tend to do what their doctors say. Better incentive designs have the potential to work, he insisted, so long as consumers are not overwhelmed. "You have to both give them tools but understand that they're not going to use tools and be as rational as you might think they would be."

DEALING WITH COMPLEX HEALTH CARE NEEDS

Gerard Anderson, professor of health policy and management and director of the Johns Hopkins Center for Hospital Finance and Management, pointed out that one important finding from health services research is that most spending and utilization are by people with complex health care needs, including people with multiple chronic conditions and/or functional limitations. For example, health services research has revealed that people with complex health care needs have much higher readmission rates on average. This finding has led to new initiatives involving clinical and community interventions, though a major challenge is finding and implementing programs that control spending while improving satisfaction and clinical outcomes.

The issues raised by people with complex health care needs run counter to the severe siloing that occurs in health care, Anderson pointed out. For example, most clinical trials exclude people with complex needs, but "they are the ones who are mostly taking the drugs." Health services research has developed approaches to fill in the missing information but not always successfully. Similarly, most fee-for-service payment systems focus on one problem at a time, though health services research has developed risk adjusters that allow for approaches like capitation. In addition, most quality metrics are disease or procedure specific, and most clinical education programs still teach about the body organ by organ. It is incumbent on health services research to break down these silos—for example, through research on care coordination.

More work is needed on adjusting outcome measures for people with chronic conditions and determining the most significant interventions and settings for people with particular sets of conditions, said Anderson. Reconciling who benefits and who pays in such situations is a critical problem, because in many cases the benefit for which an insurer pays does not occur until much later.

Anderson also took an international perspective on health services research. The United States actually uses fewer medical services than most other industrialized countries. In 2015, it had 19 percent fewer doctors, 20 percent fewer nurses, and 26 percent fewer hospital beds compared to the median country in the Organisation for Economic Co-operation and Development (OECD). However, the price of its health care makes the United States unique. This raises several new questions for health services research. For example, Anderson asked why the private sector is willing to pay 50 percent more than the public sector for the same service. One answer is that providers will spend whatever they are given, which then becomes their cost, he said. Another question is why the United States is willing to pay 50 to 100 percent more for brand name drugs than other industrialized countries. Members of Congress with whom Anderson has talked are "very concerned about this particular issue." Clearly, a research priority is making more transparent the systemic factors that shape the course of health costs and value.

Relatedly, Anderson mentioned tiered benefits in the context of pharmaceuticals. The greatest challenges for pharmaceuticals are access and adherence. Surveys by the Commonwealth Fund suggest that the US population has the most difficulty purchasing drugs among OECD countries (Sarnak et al. 2017). This finding, too, raises several compelling questions:

- How can tiered benefits be designed for very expensive drugs?
- What are the tradeoffs between who pays and who benefits?
- What can consumers understand about tier, cost, and treatment tradeoffs?

A prominent example involves hepatitis C, now responsible for the most infectious disease deaths in the United States. There are effective treatments for hepatitis C with minimal side effects, yet many people with hepatitis C are not getting care because of costs. Medicare beneficiaries must pay an average of $7,000 out of pocket, and states cannot afford to provide hepatitis C drugs to all prisoners, Medicaid recipients, and the uninsured, Anderson observed.

SUPPORTIVE AND PROTECTIVE FACTORS

Meeting participants also considered the importance of a better understanding of the protective community factors that keep people out of the health care system, such as patient health behaviors, social supports, and social services. For example, Lucy Savitz, vice president for health research for Kaiser Permanente Northwest Region, said that she helped rebuild the primary care system in Biloxi, Mississippi, after Hurricane Katrina, which impressed on her the importance of protective factors like strong social support and family cohesion. Later, at Intermountain Healthcare Institute for Healthcare Delivery Research, she observed that even people with fairly serious mental health conditions could be safely cared for in a primary care setting if they had strong social support and family cohesion.

Galea observed that research shows that one of the best ways to mitigate mental illnesses after a disaster is to focus on social support and social services. "Make sure people have houses, people have care for their elderly parents, people can get their kids into school," he said. "That mitigates the consequences on mental health." In fact, he thought it an artificial distinction to say that delivering mental health services is a health service while delivering housing is a social service. "Ultimately, they are restoring people to health or improving population health." Health services researchers are partly responsible for this, he continued, by limiting their scope to medical services and leaving other services to other people.

Westfall connected the issue to the ecology of medical care, pointing out that the 250 people each month who do not experience illness or injury is the same size as the group of people who seek medical care, but it is half the size of the group of people who experience an illness or injury but do not seek care. "Something is going on in that group that's half of the population, but they're not seeking care," he observed. "What are the factors that are occurring in the community that are protective? . . . What occurs in that box of 500 people who experience illness or injury but who don't seek care? That's a group that health services research could learn a lot from."

Ann Beal, global leader of patient solutions at Sanofi, noted that factors intrinsic to patients are also important to health care, such as patient health behaviors. "Now that we're in an era when so many of the conditions require significant patient self-management, this will help us to be much more accurate in our ability to understand not only health outcomes but also how patients then navigate the health care system." She also pointed out that, by focusing on the average, half the people are outside one standard deviation from the mean. Could a more personalized set of analyses enable health services researchers to move from observational analyses to more predictive analyses and ultimately prescriptive analysis? Anderson commented that considerable work is being done on trying to characterize people into categories in such areas as "need for social services" and "adherence to treatments." The policy challenge is that categorization tends to divide people into categories that get different levels of service.

6

DATA AND RELATED INFRASTRUCTURE NEEDS

While health services research has led to important policy changes and to improvements in health care delivery and health outcomes, and while current efforts continue to improve health care delivery, future advances will depend substantially on improving the national data infrastructure and leveraging routinely collected data. For that reason, one of the panels at the workshop considered the data infrastructure required to accelerate work on issues of quality, value, and equity in health care. The availability of exponentially more data than most envisioned a half century ago has been accompanied by the persistence of frustrating gaps, as well as formidable barriers due to technical, standards, regulatory, economic, and organizational asynchronies.

PROGRESS AND GAPS IN CLAIMS AND CLINICAL DATA

"The past decade has seen tremendous progress in assembling a data infrastructure with which to do interesting and impactful work," said Niall Brennan, president and CEO of the Health Care Cost Institute (HCCI). More data are available, and more technology is available with which to work with data, than ever before. In the past five years, CMS launched a virtual research data center that significantly lowered the cost of access to claims data and allowed smaller universities and aspiring researchers access at a price that they could afford. It switched to quarterly data refreshes instead of annual refreshes, and public use files were released that many people have found extremely useful. A new policy also enables innovators and entrepreneurs to access CMS data through the Virtual Research Data Center. The Qualified Entity Program, which also provided Medicare data to a new set of actors, required that data be combined with private sector data to improve public reporting around cost and quality.[6]

---

6 https://www.cms.gov/Research-Statistics-Data-and-Systems/Monitoring-Programs/QEMedicareData/index.html

"There are more data on Medicare beneficiaries swimming around in the health data ecosystem than ever before," he said.

At the same time, organizations like HCCI have emerged that aggregate and analyze private sector claims data and also make it available to academic researchers. HCCI has an open access data model that enables academic researchers at any university in the United States to use the data. In addition, organizations like FAIR Health and Truven Health Analytics make claims data available to researchers.

The greatest problems in leveraging data to address health care and health policy questions today, Brennan observed, are cultural rather than technological. These challenges include: (1) lack of follow through on commitments to release data; (2) legal challenges; and (3) the growth of proprietary data. Comprehensive national Medicaid data are still unavailable from CMS, despite significant time and monetary resources being devoted to a new data collection system. Medicare Advantage data exist but only one year of data is currently available to researchers.[7] "Hundreds of thousands of physicians submit hundreds of unique quality measures to CMS, but the data are not widely available," Brennan said.

Additionally, many data sets are still considered proprietary or are otherwise unavailable. For example, a Supreme Court decision has made it extremely difficult for state All Payer Claims Databases (APCDs) to incorporate all the data that they would like to incorporate because self-funded employers can no longer be legally required to contribute their data (Gobeille v. Liberty Mutual Insurance Company, 2016). Nor are data from Blue Cross Blue Shield plans systematically available to researchers. With regard to clinical data in EHRs, though progress has been made on the interoperability front, particularly as it relates to patient registry data, much of this data also remains siloed and proprietary, Brennan observed. Although claims data can be aggregated at scale and analyzed, he expressed doubts that EHR data will ever be able to achieve "universality" in the same way that claims data has.

In addition to clinical and claims data, nationally representative surveys that produce extremely valuable data continue to be cut in response to budget pressures. "We have to defend those surveys," he said. "It is easy to forget about them. They are kind of old school, because a lot of them started in the 1980s, and everybody wants to talk about big data and AI [artificial intelligence] and things like that. But if we lose things like MCBS [the Medicare Current Beneficiary Survey] or MEPS [Medical Expenditure Panel Survey] or other surveys like that, we will all be very much the worse for it."

---

7   CMS plans to release a final version of 2015 Medicare Advantage encounter data by the end of 2018. (Ravindranath, 2018)

Finally, building on points made by Blumenthal and others, and underscoring the need for changes in incentives that reward accelerating the pace of research conduct and dissemination, Brennan expanded on the point about incentives with a not entirely overstated observation that: "If you asked every health services researcher in the country what they would prefer—to be published in 18 months in the *Journal of the American Medical Association* (*JAMA*) and win an award at the [AcademyHealth Annual Research Meeting] using 10-year-old data, or to have some findings on a blog that nobody noticed but that a health care system could use to save either lives or dollars—I think the vast majority would choose *JAMA* and the AcademyHealth award because that is how their incentive structure operates."

CHALLENGE OF LINKING DATA FROM DIFFERENT SOURCES

Extending Brennan's remarks, Karl Bilimoria, a surgical oncologist and a health services and quality improvement researcher at Northwestern University's Feinberg School of Medicine and Vice President of Quality for the Northwestern Medicine health system, commented on the poor quality of data, which people are using to make important decisions. Patients are using it to decide where to go for health care. Payers are using it to decide which hospitals to direct patients and establish contracts. Hospitals are using it to set their quality targets. The problem is exemplified by the finding that the multiple public rating systems often disagree about the same hospital: one rating system may rate a certain hospital a 5 star while another rates the same hospital a 1 star. This is confusing for the end users.

He noted that currently available data used in quality measurement have some serious limitations and long delays plague the availability of data, the opportunity to use the data for change, and to monitor the results of subsequent process improvement efforts. Moreover, getting to measures that really matter is limited by the quality of the available data. While a lot of administrative data are available and are useful for measuring readmissions and mortality, they are far less useful in measuring other outcomes. Compared with chart review or clinical data, administrative data produce large numbers of false negatives and false positives. "There is miscoding in both directions that limits the validity of those data." They also are limited in doing risk adjustment, since they do not have the level of granularity needed to describe, for example, the clinical severity of the spectrum of diabetes. Yet they serve as the basis for much health care quality and public measurement systems as well as value-based purchasing systems, Bilimoria noted.

The available data are also expensive. "As somebody who writes a check for CMS data once a year, I am painfully aware," Bilimoria said. Ways to get good payer data exist and are also expensive, but CMS data are separate. Thus, there is not one place where data on all patients (all payers and ages) is easily available for quality and research uses.

On the other hand, clinical registry data can answer many clinical questions, have much more validity than administrative data, and can be extracted in a standardized fashion for quality measurement and research. But they, too, are expensive, and they typically are limited, Bilimoria noted. Due to their expense and the work required for abstraction, registries generally do not capture all the patients at a hospital, and each specialty is establishing a registry, so large hospitals are often being asked by the clinicians to participate in 50 or more different registries costing millions of dollars per year. This is likely not sustainable. The other data that are missing, Bilimoria said, are patient-reported outcomes. Everybody wants to listen to the patient, he said, "but we are far behind in being able to capture this in a standardized fashion." Greater effort is needed to move forward on these measures, he concluded, "because they do reflect the most important aspects of care to doctors and to patients."

Importantly, the future of better quality measurement requires us to much more effectively pull data directly from the EHR. This will alleviate the limitations and expense of manual abstraction. Bilimoria remarked, "While much is said of HL7 standards, natural language processing, artificial intelligence, and standardization of EHR data elements, almost no impact of this has been appreciated by the quality measurement community." Getting better data will require innovation around how the data are put in and how they are pulled out of the EHR. Quality measurement is stalled until this change can occur.

Building on earlier points made by Jack Westfall, another related issue raised by Andrew Bazemore, a practicing family physician and the director of the Robert Graham Center, was the lack of alignment between current health data infrastructure and the ecology of where patients seek and receive medical care. To demonstrate this point and its immutability over the past 50 years, Bazemore returned to the earlier cited paper by White et al. (1961) (see "Moving Research into Communities" in chapter 5). That paper "helped us to establish, in a fairly elegant way, a sense of the patient care seeking universe in the United States," said Bazemore, and that universe has not changed as much as some might think over the 50 years since.

To demonstrate this, Bazemore cited work from the Graham Center in 2001, and follow up efforts by Johansen in 2016 revealing how most care-seeking continues to occur in community and primary care settings, with very little occurring in the large academic medical centers where most training, research and data-gathering occur. (Green et al. 2001; Johansen et al. 2016). Since 1961, many new sources of data have become available, such as the Medical Expenditure Panel Survey (MEPS), the National Health Interview Survey, and data from EHRs, health information exchanges, and registries. Remarkably, said Bazemore, "the ecologies tend to map similarly over time." These efforts also point out the continued value, even in an age of myriad new data sources, of nationally representative surveys, including the MEPS from which the Ecology studies were derived. These surveys are under siege, said Bazemore, while many of the presumably richer new sources in the era of Big Data suffer proprietary lockdown, lack of sustainability models, or the inability to comment on the entire US population in a representative fashion.

That said, Bazemore noted that many new data sources are becoming available that can help to fill some of these gaps. He was particularly enthusiastic about PCORI's investment in PCORnet, a large, highly representative, national "network of networks" that collects data routinely gathered in a variety of health care settings, including hospitals, doctors' offices, and community clinics. One of its sites, the Accelerating Data Value Across a National Community Health Center Network (ADVANCE), a clinical data research network in Oregon, has even added information on the social determinants of health to the records of safety net patients on a large scale. Merging the uniform data system of community health centers with claims data would enhance understanding of the ecology of health care. For example, providers could be funded to support an upfront infrastructure that makes it easier for them to send their data to a primary care registry. Such steps would help make up for the losses of data occurring in nationally representative surveys, which, in the past, have been the main way to understand the primary care environment.

Bazemore concluded that with current advances in the national data infrastructure, it should be possible to say "that this is the county where asthma outcomes are worst, and smoking is at its highest prevalence, and here is the provider in the practice that most needs our help in caring for patients according to NHLBI guidelines for asthma action plans or smoking cessation"—a capability that the Graham Center and Community Care of North Carolina was testing 5 years ago by merging data from the state Behavioral Risk Factor Surveillance System and Medicaid to more effectively target clinicians in need of support. Yet, like many other pilots, the effort was terminated due to budget cut-backs. Additional obstacles stand in the way of such uses of data, including the limited availability of proprietary data, the sustainability of data sources, and dissemination of information and the results derived from data not only to policy makers but also to health care providers in useable ways.

COLLECTING DATA IMPORTANT TO CONSUMERS

Introducing a topic of central importance to the future of health services and systems research, Katie Martin, vice president for health policy and programs at the National Partnership for Women and Families, addressed some of the broader issues associated with data from the perspective of health care consumers. Consumers of health care have the same objectives that most stakeholders do, she said. They want a health system that keeps them healthy, that takes care of them when they are sick, and that does not threaten their financial security. However, the health care system of providers, administrators, and payers does not collect data that directly address these objectives, she pointed out. "If we were to look at the challenges of the health system from a consumer lens, it would lead us to collect a different, or maybe an additional, body of evidence."

She used alternative payment models as an example. The extent to which such models save money is an important issue, she noted, particularly if cost savings translate to lower premiums and lower cost sharing. However, the question less often asked is whether alternative payment models better meet the needs of consumers. "What do consumers want from their health care? We could use more assessment even on that basic question." Metrics might include convenient access to care, coordinated care, a trusted relationship with a provider, and care that treats patients with dignity and is consistent with their family's beliefs and goals. Once such criteria were established, alternative payment models could be measured against them and compared with fee-for-service care on these measures.

Another example involves high-deductible health plans with health savings accounts or health reimbursement arrangements. The assumption is that consumers, by having more financial risk, will express their priorities, preferences, and assessments of quality through their market power. Martin argued that a young professional who is healthy one day and diagnosed with cancer the next, or a parent whose baby was born with a congenital heart defect, does not think in these terms. These consumers of health care have considerations other than the entirely rational ones dictated by economics. Martin also suggested collecting evidence on what such products do for the costs and quality of care and the care experience.

Martin pointed out that, while the federal government is spending a great deal on health care—28 percent of federal health expenditures—US households spend just as much "and we don't think of them in the same way as we do other stakeholders" (Hartman et al. 2018). With that perspective as a lens, she had three suggestions for health services research. The first is to evaluate payment models and innovation through the additional lens of patient-centered metrics.

Such evaluations would consider such factors as health equity, meaningful patient engagement and partnership, and patient-generated information. Her second suggestion is to work on understanding the correlation between patient experiences, patient partnerships, and cost and quality outcomes. Her third suggestion is to conduct research looking at some of the foundational assumptions in health care and health financing. "What if you were to conduct [the RAND Health Insurance Experiment (Brook et al. 2006)] again in the current health care environment and with current health insurance products? Would the conclusions be the same, or would we learn some new ones about the way the world has evolved over the past 40 years? And what if we were to add racial, ethnic, and income granularity to every survey so that we can understand beyond the averages what is happening to different people across the country?"

IMPROVING DATA ACCESS, PRIVACY, AND INFRASTRUCTURE

A major topic of discussion, moderated by Adaeze Enekwechi, vice president at McDermott+Consulting and former head of health programs at the White House Office of Management and Budget, focused on the policy levers needed to make more data available and useful for accomplishing the broader goal of improving quality, access, and equity in healthcare. Brennan, who spent time as the CMS Chief Data Officer from 2010-2017, noted that "money has a tendency to solve a lot of problems." At CMS, for example, the infrastructure that provides data to researchers is a largely self-funding mechanism. A line item in the CMS budget could theoretically reduce the cost of the data to zero, though Brennan thought that charging something would inhibit frivolous uses of the data.

Continuing efforts are being made to access the data residing in EHRs, Brennan also pointed out. Upfront infrastructure funding could give providers an incentive to make their data accessible. He also mentioned the need for a "zero-tolerance policy around data blocking by either EHR vendors or individual providers and systems."

Enekwechi mentioned the possibility of combining such data with data from large surveys such as the Health and Retirement Study, which "are probably some of the best longitudinal datasets we have in the country." And Bazemore, in addition to his point about the need to create uniform data reporting systems to gather data from rural primary health clinics, spoke to the potential of bringing informaticists and clinicians together to design systems based on patient-centered outcome questions. Such systems could incorporate information about the social determinants of health and provide an opportunity "to use clinical data merged across multiple levels—inpatient, outpatient, laboratory, and community—to understand how we need to risk adjust and adapt to the social drivers of health care."

The discussion also focused on privacy issues. Brennan commented that maintaining privacy is critically important. However, he also made the point that the Health Insurance Portability and Accountability Act (HIPAA) is, in fact, a permissive regulation that is often misinterpreted by nonresearchers to block data sharing. Further, he noted that there are methods that allow for statistical deidentification while maintaining the utility of the data. With use of the appropriate security protocols, "you can do a lot and not worry that you are compromising or threatening people's privacy." However, other workshop participants countered that fears of how the data might be misused and other privacy concerns are legitimate barriers to sharing and worthy of attention. One proposed approach was a model policy that would provide health care entities with a safe harbor in case of a data breach if they followed all of the HIPAA requirements and other relevant guidance. Resolving these issues is core to the transformative progress of health system research and improvement.

The discussion then broadened to a consideration of public health data and data on the social determinants of health, including the possibility of a "meaningful use revolution in the public health sector to tie those data together." For example, data on both the social service and health care needs of an individual could help determine whether more money spent on social services could reduce health care spending. Martin pointed out that this kind of work is going on at the federal level, but the social determinants data are receiving less emphasis than the clinical data, and "there is opportunity to encourage the administration to accelerate those data elements and data collections."

Ultimately, as several participants noted, the most critical step to promoting policy changes to improve the data infrastructure and data access is demonstrating the value in leveraging data to end users, including health care consumers, clinicians, health systems leaders, payers, and policy makers. Without first demonstrating value and creating demand, it will continue to be challenging to address the cultural barriers mentioned by the panelists.

7

PRIORITIES FROM USER PERSPECTIVES

Virtually every sector in the nation is, directly or indirectly, a significant stakeholder in the future of health services research. Meeting participants and discussants, including, in particular, those from the policy, consumer, clinician, and payer communities, discussed priorities for the field of health services research over the next decade. These discussions highlighted important research priorities for improving health and health care outcomes as well as priorities for improving the infrastructure needed to support and transform health services research. A consistent theme was the importance of focusing on implementation science as core among the challenges and opportunities.

PRIORITIES FROM A POLICY MAKER'S PERSPECTIVE

Charles (Chip) Kahn, president and chief executive officer of the Federation of American Hospitals, identified four areas of health services research relevant to both policy and practice: coverage, quality, accountability, and transparency. Using that lens, he articulated three research priorities for the field.

First, Kahn commented that health services research has not been very successful in helping policy makers move away from fee-for-service and that, therefore, it is critically important to understand the impact of alternative payment models on health outcomes. The greatest successes remain the Social Security Amendments of 1983 and the diagnosis-related group codes. The Medicare Access and Children's Health Insurance Program Reauthorization Act of 2015 "shows that there is a lot of work to do," according to Kahn. "Rather than value-based purchasing—because I don't know what value really is—I'd say we need results-based purchasing, and the field needs to tell us and guide policy makers as to what that ought to be." A number of natural experiments are taking place, such as those presented by differences in coverage between California and Texas. "We need to understand that better," he said, particularly "the policy implications." Whatever payment models are developed, they need to incorporate risk adjustment and socioeconomic disparities, he added. As previously mentioned, health services research also needs to incorporate broader social issues such as loneliness, he pointed out.

Second, while the field of health services research has done a good job of producing measures both of quality and performance, Kahn commented that there is a need for additional research that demonstrates which quality measures are critical to improving outcomes. "But we have a Tower of Babel here," he said. Many measures have been produced and used, and many measures are required by payers, "but I would argue that we don't really understand which measures are successful in moving the dial. We don't have a good way of assessing gaps and then figuring out how to fill them."

Finally, he noted that big data and artificial intelligence are going to enhance care, with both the public sector and academia moving forward in these areas. But even if some analytics are great, not all will lead to improvements, and, in fact, some may result in harm. Also, data analytics are going to influence policies regarding payment, accountability, and transparency in currently unknown ways. "It's essential that the understanding of the implications of these new analytics be well understood," he said. "Frankly, those who are producing them and doing great work are not the people necessarily to answer that question." While heavy regulation is not the answer, the field needs to look at this issue from a broad perspective and make recommendations so that policy makers can understand and respond appropriately, he said. "We have to figure out how to make analytics work for patients [and] caregivers and at the same time figure out how that is also going to work in a policy context."

PRIORITIES FROM A CLINICIAN'S PERSPECTIVE

William Bornstein, system chief medical officer and chief quality and patient safety officer for Emory Healthcare and professor of medicine in the Emory University School of Medicine, took a more granular approach by discussing what he needs to take care of patients. Type 2 diabetes encapsulates many of the challenges he and other providers face. Patients, family members, and health care providers have a belief that diabetes is brought on by inactivity and obesity, although genetic and biological factors are obviously also involved. This belief can lead providers and family members to conclude that people with diabetes either do not understand that lifestyle changes can ameliorate the disease or are not motivated to change. In reality, these patients do understand and are extraordinarily motivated to change, said Bornstein. "We fail them in this regard by not being able to help them."

He also pointed out that the social determinants of health contribute to diabetes. Patients who live in food deserts or in neighborhoods where it is unsafe to walk face challenges in changing their behavior, "but honestly I don't find that my more affluent patients are having tremendous success in this regard." The barriers appear to be ubiquitous, which calls for a much better understanding than exists today of how providers can help patients change their behavior.

These issues are not unique to diabetes, leading Bornstein to suggest three research priorities for the field of health services research moving forward. The first is the need to understand the levers for behavior change. "Intuition in this regard is usually dead wrong," he said, "and the usual incentives that we think motivate human behavior really are not fully explanatory." Behavioral economics has provided some insight into how people change, including the idea that their behavior can be "nudged" through subtle messages, but this research is still in its early stages.

The second priority is to deal more effectively with overburden and burnout among providers. "If providers are suffering, we can't effectively or optimally relieve the suffering of our patients," Bornstein said. New care models may reduce the burden on providers. Additionally, electronic health records had great promise, but that promise has not been realized, Bornstein said. Providers still need better and more effective decision support. Furthermore, new kinds of errors are occurring that would not be occurring in the absence of these systems. "We need more research in terms of how we optimize clinical decision support and how we reduce overburden that's coming directly from the confinements that EHRs have been designed with."

Finally, building on earlier points raised by Katie Martin, Bornstein mentioned that the financial risk of care has been changing. "It's shifting to providers, it's shifting to patients. There are undesirable consequences of that, and there are desirable consequences. Behavioral economics can help us understand how more effectively to mitigate those undesirable consequences while retaining the benefits."

Related to these research priorities raised by Bornstein, earlier comments from Gerard Anderson highlight the importance of future research focused on determining the most effective models of managing the challenges of high-need, high-cost patients. Robert Phillips, vice president of research and policy at the American Board of Family Medicine and adjunct faculty at Georgetown University and Virginia Commonwealth University, also suggested that there was a need for more research focused on understanding how to identify protective community factors, health risks, and resources for patients and communities before patients become high-need. One way to do this is to learn more about managing the interfaces of the ecology of medical care boxes, as mentioned by

Jack Westfall and Andrew Bazemore earlier in the workshop. How can home health care change to do things that hospitals used to do? How can patients transition into primary care to keep them from coming back to the hospital? Work at the whole-person and whole-community levels can yield more progress than carving up problems by organ system or disease, he said.

PRIORITIES FROM A CONSUMER ADVOCATE'S PERSPECTIVE

The American Association of Retired Persons (AARP) uses health services research to understand the impact of policies or interventions on consumers, observed Lina Walker, vice president of health security in AARP's Public Policy Institute. It also uses health services research to engage with consumers and help them make better decisions about their health and well-being. With this background, she highlighted several research priorities for the field as well as several approaches for improving the infrastructure available to support health services research.

One area in which health services research falls short is in its treatment of the social determinants of health. Researchers typically rely on ZIP codes or dual status (Medicare-Medicaid beneficiaries) to estimate social determinants, but these are not sufficient as proxies, Walker said. "Social determinants include transportation, food and security, housing, income, social connectedness, and I would argue . . . that ZIP codes and dual status barely capture any of those factors." A cross-cutting conversation is needed, she said, about how to capture, collect, and integrate data on social determinants with claims and clinical data.

The second point she made is that health services research needs to understand how to capture and reflect the value that consumers place on their choices. For example, convenience is a powerful factor among the people AARP represents. When people are moving into a nursing home, they want to find a facility that is convenient to family and friends. "Those considerations are very much a part of health care decision making. They are not outside the realm of health, and for those reasons, they have to be reflected in health services research."

She pointed out that health services research has two obligations: to identify and focus on the issues that matter most, and to provide the information that helps people make informed decisions. A more expansive scope of health services research would advance human health and well-being by integrating and assessing across systems.

Related to this, David Balch, of the Patient Advocate Foundation, noted the importance of understanding the "financial toxicity" associated with shifting health care costs to patients. When patients have excessive medical bills, they begin skipping meals, rent payments, utility payments, and car payments, but, eventually, they hit a "breaking point" that affects their medical care. "One way that health services research could intervene on behalf of those patients is to figure out how to have a conversation early and often about those areas and figure out what interventions can help patients manage those aspects of financial toxicity."

Finally, Walker noted that readmissions and death are outcomes often used to reflect health care quality, but these are not necessarily the outcomes that are most important to patients. She told of a conversation with a car service driver who was in constant pain from neck surgery. A quality measure that considers only readmissions would miss his problems. The quandary is that not enough evidence is available to develop such a measure, but the lack of a measure makes it hard to develop the evidence. "How do we break that cycle?" How do we assess care match with patient goals? Some Medicaid programs and health systems are developing their own measures and evaluations, though they may not be published. Some systems have employed more patient-reported outcomes or have tried to incorporate values in decision making. Walker noted that in order to move the science and improve care, it is important to continue to support the development of and share information about patient-centered outcomes that measure health care quality from the patient and family perspective.

PRIORITIES FROM A PAYER'S PERSPECTIVE

Mary Applegate, medical director for the Ohio Department of Medicaid, noted that the field of health services research is ripe for disruption, and this observation led to her recommendations for research and infrastructure-related priorities over the next decade.

First, building on earlier themes, Applegate commented on the misalignment of incentives in academia that were previously mentioned by Blumenthal and Ferris (see Applying Health Services Research in Practice and Policy, chapter 3) - incentives which focus on publication and promotion, and do not lead to generation of the type of evidence that is needed by payers. "What I need in the Medicaid program is an inch deep and a mile wide, because, in Ohio, I have three million people I need to take care of." On a related note, Applegate highlighted the need for incentives that encourage researchers to focus on implementation science. She pointed out that there are effective models by which payers can partner with academic researchers. For instance, academic medical centers can work with an honest broker who could be contacted by payers when they have an outstanding question that could be addressed through health services research.

The honest broker could then identify an academic medical center with the expertise and the data needed to address the question. In Ohio, Applegate has established an honest broker system that enables her to work closely with academic researchers on implementation issues.

Applegate also argued that there is a need for research that can be completed faster in order to inform critical health policy decisions. As an example, she stated that more than 4,000 people are dying in Ohio every year for reasons related to opioid use. "I need to know with predictive modeling who is at risk for misuse, dependency, overdose, and death—those are four different endpoints—and we need to know at the point in service what the deal is so that it can shape my conversation at the time that I'm actually seeing the patient." This is already possible with infant mortality, she noted, where the EHR can provide information about who is at risk for preterm birth and whose babies are at a greater risk for infant mortality. When patients hear that their babies are at risk, they do things differently.

Applegate also highlighted the importance of designing payment policies and health care systems that engender trust. In order to do this, she pointed out that the outcome measures used by health services researchers should be coproduced by researchers, patients, and clinicians to ensure that they are relevant to end-users. Indeed, the need is so great that her system has been producing such measures on its own. The problem is that different states have created measures that are similar but not the same, "which means we haven't capitalized on what health services research can actually do for us. This is a plea to please work directly with the people who are going to be using the results of the research."

In general, greater cooperation and standardization among the states could lead to faster improvement in each of the states, she said. For example, some standardization of evaluation across states would be "a whole lot better than what we have now, which is an evaluation state by state." Cooperation among states could help build links between clinical practice and public health. Standardization also could increase collaboration among private sector efforts to harness EHR data for health services research.

Other participants highlighted the importance of understanding the impact of provider consolidation on health disparities and other health outcomes and of establishing better measures for value in health care since prevailing measures were developed based on the current fee-for-service payment structure.

Applegate concluded by pointing out that innovation is fun. For example, she raised the question of whether it would be possible to use block chain technology to link datasets without having to worry about privacy concerns, and the impact of such a system on value-based purchasing. These types of innovations will require partnerships, including partnerships with information technologists, educators, and patients, as well as a focus on implementation science. Such partnerships represent a new way of operating, she concluded, but the information they generate can improve health and save lives.

CROSS-CUTTING NATIONAL PRIORITY: LEVERAGING DATA

Drawing on conversations from earlier panels as well as the discussion that ensued following the presentations of stakeholder specific priorities for the field of health services research, additional themes emerged. The first relates to the need for organizations to cooperate in sharing and assessing the data essential to health services research, and the second relates to the need for a national conversation regarding the ultimate goals of the health care system: the focus on health.

Regarding data sharing, participants considered the prospects for pooling data from different health systems to answer questions in health services research and about health systems performance. Bornstein expressed the view that "the patients we serve and the citizens of this country are supportive of more access to this kind of data. The barriers seem to be more at the level of legislation and regulation." Also, when issues are raised about privacy, managers tend to shy away from data sharing out of concerns about potential HIPAA violations. However, HIPAA is relatively permissive, Bornstein said, reiterating a point Brennan made earlier. "We need to take stronger positions on these things. We can do more under today's regulatory environment, but I would [also] like to see the regulations and legislation change."

Kahn referred to the possibility of technological solutions to the problem. Again, reiterating earlier points made by Brennan, Kahn noted that technologic advances allow for data deidentification in ways that both prevent reidentification and preserve the utility of the data. However, these advances may not solve the policy problems, because "privacy is the kind of area where the few, not the many, make policy."

Walker suggested the need for funding streams that require collaboration among diverse stakeholders, which would provide incentives for sharing data. On this issue, Rainu Kaushal, of Weill Cornell Medicine, noted that several of the academic medical centers in New York City have been sharing data through PCORnet. "The tools are out there," she said. "It's the political and cultural issues" that are preventing more widespread data sharing. Joe Selby of PCORI noted that he sees clinical data being combined with health plan enrollment data or Medicaid enrollment data in individual projects, but not more widely. "If all the parties become interested, if there is something in it for everybody, it will happen," he said. "But I haven't seen anything yet to make me optimistic."

Darshak Sanghavi, of OptumLabs, commented on the large number of data-pooling activities taking place in the private sector. The resulting data are typically proprietary but are often available for researchers. Applegate agreed and noted that private industry usually has health researchers embedded within their own organizations to understand these data. "Is there a way to have a virtual community so that we have methods and some standardization so that we can better understand what's going on?" she asked. "That's a challenge for the field." Added Kahn: "We have to figure out the best way to make that world work, because we're a commercial country, and this is going to be commercial at the end of the day."

CROSS-CUTTING NATIONAL PRIORITY: FOCUS ON HEALTH

With regard to the second theme, Sandro Galea stated that "we are long overdue for a national conversation about what we're trying to do" in health care. If the goal of US health care is to have people die healthy, so that morbidity at the end of life is compressed, different decisions would be made about public- and private-sector research and development. "If it's true that we're trying to each live the longest possible life as healthy as possible, then it changes a lot of what we do. It changes a lot of the questions we ask. It changes what we invest in. [But] I don't think we've had a national conversation." On a related note, Gerard Anderson observed that the underlying factors that influence health raise very broad issues for health services research.

Michael Chernew pointed to the inevitable complications raised by the extensive cross-subsidization that occurs in the health care system. This feature of the system raises questions about authority, about who is going to do what, and about how much one group should pay for benefits, such as convenience, that flow to other groups. Some of these questions could be answered by policy makers trying to foresee the future of health care needs in the United States. For example, as more care is delivered in outpatient facilities and as technology progresses, health services research will need to change its areas of emphasis. However, that can be difficult, given the unpredictability of the changes going on in the health care system. In general, Chernew argued that policy makers should try to have a "soft touch" on delivery systems to allow maximum flexibility. "If you could give a broad set of parameters about quality and spending and allow the delivery systems and organizations to innovate underneath that, I think you'd be better off than if you tried to prescribe very specific ways in which organizations have to produce care with very specific types of resources."

This observation led to a discussion of the influence of health services research on the health care system. One way of looking at the field's history is to conclude that influential papers have not always affected policy in a meaningful way. However, participants objected to that interpretation, pointing to, for example, the ways in which health services research affected the adoption of accountable care organizations or section 2713 of the Patient Protection and Affordable Care Act, covering preventive health services. In some cases, health services research has simply moved the conversation in particular directions, but in other cases, such as through the work on checklists and patient activation (Hales and Pronovost, 2006), health services research has had a direct impact on health care. Furthermore, as Anderson pointed out, it takes time for research to make its way into practice in health care.

As an extension of these themes, the panelists discussed the possibility of organizations that normally compete with each other collaborating to set priorities on issues that are important to them all in improving the health of their clients and populations. Focusing specifically on funders of health services research, Timothy Ferris, of the Massachusetts General Physicians Organization, noted that funders often differentiate themselves by looking for the next "great idea, and maybe that's a luxury that we can't afford." Kahn noted that legislation sets priorities for many federal agencies, which limits their ability to establish their own priorities. Instead, the private sector, including foundations, may need to engage in priority-setting processes while the government "can do what it can do." However, Walker pointed out that legislation is not necessarily an obstacle. "There's always room to maneuver," she said. "These are all overlapping sets of priorities."

Finally, participants noted the importance of ensuring that the field of health services research communicates and demonstrates its value in the design of successful policies and in the improvement of health and health care outcomes. On a related note, several workshop participants commented on the need for health services research to make its work and findings more accessible to nonspecialists, people "sitting around their kitchen tables." For example, Enekwechi cited a recent project she conducted on improving birth outcomes through payment policy levers in which the language of health services research and payment policies was less well understood by some of the stakeholders. "Health services researchers talk to each other, but we don't translate very well."

8

RESEARCH FOR A TWENTY-FIRST-CENTURY HEALTH SYSTEM

To pursue the priorities identified over the course of the meeting, the summary session discussion focused on approaches to strengthen the field as a transformational force for a twenty-first-century health system. "What would the headlines from 2025 look like if these deliberations had a successful outcome?" asked Jonathan Perlin, president of clinical services and chief medical officer at Health Corporation of America and moderator of the session. Would they be:

- Health policy is routinely driven by evidence on system performance;
- Data derived from the care experience provides a ubiquitous utility for learning and improvement;
- Health services research is the engine that drives continuous learning and improved decision-making;
- Health innovations are assessed in real-time; or
- Research on health services and systems performance spans both care and health?

ISSUE: CONCEPTS AND GOALS

Perlin noted the need for "a concept of operations for a twenty-first-century approach to health services research." Such a concept may start with a research agenda, but it also includes how that agenda is used and which constituents are involved. It involves articulating a value proposition for each constituency, which, in turn, raises the question of the "financial ecology" that makes research possible. The interface between research infrastructure and practice application must be as seamless as possible.

With respect to developing a research agenda, and building on themes from the previous chapter, Andrew Bindman, professor of medicine, epidemiology, and biostatistics at the University of California, San Francisco, commented that the health services research community needs clearer goals—either a shared goal or a limited set of goals. Its goals cannot be simply a description of what health services researchers do or how they do it. Rather, researchers need to be clear and specific in saying what they are applying themselves to do. A lack of clarity regarding goals and responsibilities is one reason why some in Congress ask if there is redundancy in the system, he pointed out. The leaders of public agencies are well positioned to observe, broker, and articulate the field's goals.

Additionally, Bindman remarked that since, in a political process, focus and priorities are determined by the consensus of end users and stakeholders, the health services research community cannot be the only keepers of their shared goals. Instead, influential stakeholders need to share, support, and participate in achieving these goals. In particular, public investment can engage and organize private partnerships directed toward shared goals. On a related note, Lee Fleisher, professor of anesthesiology and medicine at the University of Pennsylvania Perelman School of Medicine, pointed out that breaking down silos is an interesting issue in a medical world of specialties. It is particularly interesting, he said, in the context of mental health and the ongoing opioid epidemic, where "the inability to get data even from our insurance companies around mental health issues is a huge stumbling block." Great opportunities exist, but taking advantage of those opportunities requires getting all the stakeholders in a single room to talk with each other. Even greater opportunities would be available by taking advantage of the changes going on in the insurance industry and the retail industry that are changing the way people interact with these businesses. Fleisher raised the issue of how health services research should interface with chief executive officers and the overall architecture of the health system, including academic centers and community centers.

To ensure that the goals articulated as part of the research agenda are accomplished, many participants called for better coordination of the federal investment in the field. A growing number of funders, including AHRQ, PCORI, NIH, Center for Medicare & Medicaid Innovation, and the VA, have demonstrated "a marvelous spirit of curiosity in the field of health services research," said Bindman. These entities cooperate and interact with one another, but they do not have a formal process to make decisions in an efficient and coherent manner. "This has left us vulnerable to questions of whether our approach is redundant and inefficient." A common or collaborative governance/coordination structure could help to enhance alignment among agencies around a shared set of goals for the field of health services research. "A city the size of health services research needs a planning commission to sort out its investment and a growth strategy guided by its goals," Bindman concluded. "The White House budget has proposed some ways of reorganizing these investments . . . I see this as a symptom of leaving ourselves vulnerable to addressing fundamental questions about our shared goals and the best way to organize ourselves to achieve them. I think this meeting has helped us to start that conversation, but we have substantial work to do to give our field the infrastructure it needs. And judging by the White House policy, which has called for reorganizing AHRQ into NIH for two years in a row, the clock is ticking."

In addition to improving coordination and governance among federal funders of health services research, Robert Phillips, from the American Board of Family Medicine, pointed out that health services research is being done in many buckets across private and public agencies. There is a need to improve coordination not just among federal agencies but also among federal agencies and private and non-profit organizations. If the field is spending $5 billion in total, could it get more value from that expenditure, Phillips asked.

Bindman also noted that the governance or coordination structure that is created should be informed by a set of metrics, plotted against time toward its goals, which will create a system of accountability and support communication within and outside of the community about what the field of health services research has accomplished. A low-level metric might be directed toward a specific problem, "but at some point we need to evolve past that and demonstrate real impact on a population level." Public investments can help develop these metrics, collect the necessary information, report on the results over time, and make an evidence-based case for the return on investment. This can then help guide the amount of funding and whether it should grow over time. Shorter-term metrics may also be helpful in guiding policy decision-makers and other essential stakeholders contending with immediate challenges.

With respect to shared goals, participants called for a national conversation about the outcomes the health care system is working to achieve, and the proportion of health services research that should be focused on macro-level policy questions versus micro-level questions focused on individual health systems, hospitals, or clinics. Participants also supported the development of new models of funding and new research methods that allow for rapid cycle research to inform policy makers as well as for funding to support implementation science. In addition to rethinking funding models, another theme from the meeting was the incentives in academia, which focus on publication and promotion rather than on developing the evidence that is most important to end users. Considering ways to restructure these incentives to reward research that changes practices, even if only on a small scale, could promote greater interaction between evidence producers and evidence users and more impactful health services research.

The ability of the field to address research priorities and impact health care and policy and to leverage recent advances in data analytics, including predictive analytics and artificial intelligence, would be enhanced if health care and patient-generated data were routinely shared and leveraged to address problems within the health care system and community settings. Also key to progress on these goals is enhanced interaction among health system leaders, policy makers and health services researchers. However, as various participants noted, there are a number of cultural and policy barriers that prevent the sharing of data on a national level to support health services research, clinical research, and continuous learning. These include, for example, the growth of proprietary data, concerns about privacy protections, the lack of follow-through on commitments to share data, and the inability to integrate community and social determinants data with health care data.

On the data issue, Richard Besser of the Robert Wood Johnson Foundation (RWJF), underscored the importance of strategies to ensure linkage of health care data with community and social determinants data, such as housing, education, and transportation, observing that "if you are not able to include these issues in the datasets you are analyzing, you are going to be missing a critical barrier to health." On a related note, participants discussed the need to maintain investments in nationally representative surveys, which also contain valuable data for addressing important health care and health policy questions. Addressing these barriers will require a sustained national effort that engages stakeholders from across the health care sector as well as from other sectors of society that have a direct impact on health such as housing, transportation, and education.

ISSUE: COMMUNICATING VALUE FOR PATIENTS AND SOCIETY

Ultimately, in order to demonstrate the importance of continued federal investment in health services research, numerous participants across both days of the symposium commented on the need for the field to better articulate its value in terms of improving health, health care, and health policy. Part of demonstrating value requires ensuring that the results and benefits of health services research are available to all potential end users. It also requires developing a communication strategy, which may include changing the name of the field so that it is more intuitive to end users, and improving the translation of results from health services research to drive changes in health care, communities, and federal and local policies.

On this point, Ellie Dehoney, vice president of public policy and programs at Research!America, argued that health services research needs to be described in compelling terms. For example: "If you don't use it, our fiscal crisis is going to get worse, people are going to die, and neither of those things need to happen." It should not be the fourth kind of research that is considered but the first, "because medical research makes no sense if it isn't disseminated in a way that reaches every American and helps with their health."

As stated by Perlin, "if that market isn't calling, how do we strengthen the articulation of the value proposition and therefore strengthen the market?" Focusing on public investments in health services research, Phillips remarked that the relative growth in funding for health services research has not kept up with the growth in biomedical research funding. Yet, with respect to the gap between knowledge and delivery, the need for health services research is even more pressing than it has been in the past. To support the need for additional and continued federal support, the field needs to better communicate its value and develop a process for sharing results.

Building on this theme, Besser stated that "One of the things I found in my eight years [as health and medical editor] at ABC [News] is that, for most people in health and in science, communication is an afterthought." However, from his perspective, the "work begins after the research is completed," he added. A paper may provide evidence, but that evidence then needs to be turned into programs that lead to change in communities, "so that you are not writing that same paper five to ten years later because nothing has changed." Though some progress has been made with this issue, a communication strategy could further improve understanding of the value proposition for health services research and make policy makers more aware of the field.

Bindman commented that, in order to demonstrate value, it is critical to ensure that the benefits of health services research are available to all and not just to the organizations and entities that have private resources to access those benefits. He also suggested that there ought to be separate funding mechanisms to support innovation, evaluation, and implementation within the field of health services research, as the appropriate funding mechanisms for these three areas of research are likely to be very different. Building on earlier themes from the conference, Bindman pointed out that implementation science, in particular, has lagged behind, in part because funding mechanisms used to determine internal validity are not necessarily suited for strategies to implement what works. Similarly, Fleisher commented that the field needs "to be more inventive about funding strategies to support implementation." Accomplishing this requires thinking about the incentive structure for new health services researchers needed to support implementation science. Traditional research that is published in the *New England Journal of Medicine* and *JAMA* is the usual way to move up the academic ladder, but implementation science, despite interest among health system leaders and young researchers, is more difficult to get funded and published in highly visible journals, said Fleisher.

In addition to novel funding mechanisms, Phillips remarked that, in order to inform change in care delivery, the field must develop new methods of research, find value in current research—including negative findings—and share successes and failures more widely and thoroughly than is done today. Clear needs exist for more high-risk funding, more innovation, more translation, greater speed, greater pragmatism, and the integration of social services into health services research.

Addressing the particular importance of positioning health services research as a more routine and integral component of the delivery process, Perlin raised a number of additional questions for consideration, including:

- How can research be best integrated into care?
- What sort of research can be supported by health systems, and what do health systems and providers need to learn?
- Are there vehicles to make system-specific learning transportable, scalable, and networked so that the learning process can be accelerated?
- What are the roles of professionals, professional organizations, and organizations outside of health care systems and academic institutions in supporting this work?
- How can the best research investments be identified?
- What are the synergies that enhance value between federal investment, private investment, and the work that health systems are doing?
- How can health services research move beyond the walls of the institution and incorporate the ubiquitous determinants of health?

An overriding theme from this session was that the field of health services research needs to determine how to effectively engage both across the field and with end users to break down silos and demonstrate value. Conversations with end users, including Congressional representatives, need to describe the problems facing the health care system and how health services research can and is helping to solve those problems. As suggested by Fleisher, there is also a need to determine how to most appropriately engage patients to inform future priorities and goals for the field of health services research.

ISSUE: MOBILIZING FOR TRANSFORMATION

The field of health services research has led to important insights and advances in health care policy and health care quality, delivery, and efficiency, ultimately improving patient care and outcomes. However, many outstanding issues remain. Over the course of the symposium, participants discussed many health and health care challenges and opportunities for which the evidence need is pressing, including those related to: engaging the social determinants of health; addressing overburden and burnout among clinicians; determining effective alternative payment models; developing approaches for integrating genetics and related knowledge about individual patient variation into the care process; engineering health care systems so that they result in the most effective care for patients; understanding how to better address the needs of high-need, high-cost patients; building the capacity to take advantage of technologies for patient- and family-activated home and remote site health and health care services.

While raising macro-level issues such as strategic coordination of research agendas and improving the national infrastructure for a fully interoperable health information system, participants emphasized various emerging strategic field focus priorities for the next decade, including:

- structured approaches to assessing, applying, and adapting the delivery system to insights and tools related to precision medicine;
- system strategies for ensuring patient safety in the face of an increasingly complex diagnostic and treatment environment;
- embedding health services research skills and tools into care delivery as a basic component of a continuously learning health system;
- establishing reliable data from the routine care experience as a secure utility enhancing evidence development, predictive modeling, and continuous care improvement;
- incorporating necessary demographic, environmental, social, and community data as an integral component of that data utility;
- devising and demonstrating the impact of innovative payment and care delivery models for improving system performance and population health;
- identification and application of quality assessment metrics that are most reliable at gauging system-wide performance in delivering care and improving health;
- positioning patient and family involvement, interests, priorities, and data as a central resource for care design and assessment;

- developing the full and effective use of artificial intelligence and machine learning as transformational resources for knowledge development and services improvement; and
- effective approaches to translating and scaling research insights, including effective expression of the consequences of inaction.

The range of the issues is so substantial that relying on spontaneous and sometimes serendipitous response capacity in the field will not meet the need. Rather, a deliberate and coordinated set of activities is required to prepare—to transform—the field. In effect, participants individually and collectively presented a call to action for the field to mobilize sustained initiatives to:

- expand the **vision** to account for the full range of health system forces in play;
- develop a robust taxonomy of the issue and leverage **priorities** for action;
- identify the **tools and strategies**—available and emerging—to refine and deploy in the change process;
- steward the societal-wide advancement of a **culture of continuous learning** and sharing throughout the system;
- foster the development of the **data infrastructure and research teams** required for real-time insights and feedback in the virtuous cycle of continuous learning;
- create a working **network of stakeholders,** including patients as partners in research, for expedited coordination, collaboration, and, as required, governance;
- establish shared network-wide **goals** and a process for tracking and adapting strategies;
- characterize the anticipated and actual **results** for improvement, in qualitative and quantitative personal, societal, and economic terms;
- **link** those real and potential returns to investments and investment requirements among stakeholders—federal and nonfederal; and
- capture and **communicate** the contributions, real and potential, in a broad, visible, and deliberate campaign.

Accomplishing such an agenda will require continued engagement and conversations among evidence producers and evidence users as well as greater collaboration and articulation of research priorities among federal and nonfederal funders of health services research. Underscored was the potential to position the NAM meeting and conversation as starting point for a national conversation about the future of the field because the health services research field is ripe for disruption. Lisa Simpson, from AcademyHealth, stated that "we are at a pivotal time in thinking about federal support for health services research. . . . There is a policy window of opportunity that is opening." As the field moves forward and federal programs are reauthorized, eliminated, or transformed, plentiful opportunities will arise to create something "new, different, more responsive."

The critical policy window, combined with the outstanding issues within the United States health care system, present an important opportunity for the field of health services research to articulate its priority and demonstrate its utility. Richard Besser highlighted the need for the field to focus on action. Better health in America, from the local to the national level, requires the contributions of health services research, and, in order to promote action, it is necessary for the field of health services research to work with people in other sectors to bring their methods to bear on broader questions about health and well-being.

"We want to understand how the health care system fits into the broader picture," he concluded. Health services researchers "are the ones who can help answer that question." In addition, Carolyn Clancy and Andrew Bindman commented that decision makers and policy makers do not generally have the luxury to wait for perfect health services research. Instead, they need to act with whatever information they have, and the health services research community needs to be responsive to this. Providing those quick returns can build credibility for health services research, so that clients know researchers can provide value in building toward longer-term goals.

In the final analysis, capturing the insights, opportunities, and obligations identified during this National Academy of Medicine meeting will require sustained and deliberate conversations involving stakeholders from throughout the nation. Those conversations have started, but achieving their potential for impact will require commitment and active involvement in the years ahead from the organizations represented at the meeting, not only on their own behalf, but as recruiters, motivators, and engagers of public and private stakeholders across the nation. Congress has recently made available resources and a mandate to study future federal funding in the field. This NAM meeting and publication can serve as a reference and foundation for that work. The physical and financial health of the nation is at stake.

REFERENCES

Agency for Healthcare Research and Quality. 2018 August 1. Mission and Budget. Retrieved from: https://ahrq.gov/cpi/about/mission/index.html.

Bindman, A. 2013. The evolution of health services research. *Health Services Research* 48(2):349-353.

Brook, R. H., E. B. Keeler, K. N. Lohr, J. P. Newhouse, J. E. Ware, W. H. Rogers, A. R. Davies, C. D. Sherbourne, G. A. Goldberg, P. Camp, C. Kamberg, A. Leibowitz, J. Keesey, and D. Reboussin. 2006. The Health Insurance Experiment: A classic RAND study speaks to the current health care reform debate. Santa Monica, CA: RAND Corporation. Available at: http://www.rand.org/content/dam/rand/pubs/research_briefs/2006/RAND_RB9174.pdf

Chernew, M. E., M. R. Shah, A. Wegh, S. N. Rosenberg, I. A. Juster, A. B. Rosen, M. C. Sokol, K. Yu-Isenberg, and A. M. Fendrick. 2008. Impact of decreasing copayments on medication adherence within a disease management program. *Health Affairs* 27(1):103-112.

Desai, S., L. A. Hatfield, A. L. Hicks, M. E. Chernew, and A. Mehrotra. 2016. Association between availability of a price transparency tool and outpatient spending. *JAMA* 315(17):1874-1881.

Eisenberg, J. M., and E. J. Power. 2000. Transforming insurance coverage into quality health care: voltage drops from potential to delivered quality. *JAMA* 284(16):2100-2107.

Folsom Group. 2012. Communities of solution: the Folsom Report revisited. *Annals of Family Medicine* 10(3):250-260.

Folsom, M. 1967. *Health is a Community Affair*. NCCHS. Cambridge, MA: Harvard University Press.

Frank, M. B., J. Hsu, M. B. Landrum, and M. E. Chernew. 2015. The impact of a tiered network on hospital choice. *Health Services Research* 50(5):1628-1648.

Gobeille v. Liberty Mutual Insurance Company. 577 U.S. _ (2016).

Gold, M. R. 2016. Critical challenges in making health services research relevant to decision makers. *Health Services Research* 51(1):9-15.

Green, L.A., G.E. Fryer Jr., B.P. Yawn, D. Lanier, and S.M. Dovey. 2001. The ecology of medical care revisited. New England Journal of Medicine 344:2021-2025.

Hales, B. M., and P. J. Pronovost. 2006. The checklist—a tool for error management and performance improvement. *Journal of Critical Care* 21(3):231-5.

Hartman, M., A. B. Martin, N. Espinosa, and A. Catlin. 2018. The National Health Expenditure Accounts Team. National Health Care Spending In 2016: Spending And Enrollment Growth Slow After Initial Coverage Expansions. Health Affairs (Millwood) 37(1):150-160.

IOM (Institute of Medicine). 1979. *Health Services Research: Report of a Study.* Washington, DC: National Academy of Sciences.

Johansen, M. E., S. M. Kircher, and T. R. Huerta. 2016. Reexamining the ecology of medical care. *New England Journal of Medicine* 374(5):495-496.

Kaushal, R. 2018. Pending Citation.

Keyes, K. M., and S. Galea. 2016. *Population Health Science.* New York: Oxford University Press.

Labarraque, A.G. 1829. Instructions and observations regarding the use of the chlorides of soda and lime. In: Porter J, editor. New Haven, CT: Baldwin and Treadway.

Lind, J. 1753. Treatise of the Scurvy. Edinburgh: Sands, Murray, and Cochran.

Lohr, K., and D. Steinwachs. 2002. "Health services research: an evolving definition of the field." *Health Services Research* 37(1):7-9.

McGinnis, J.M. 2018. *Introductory Remarks.* Presentation at the National Academy of Medicine Symposium on Building the Evidence Base for Improving Health Care, 27 February 2018. National Academy of Medicine, Washington, DC.

Mongan, J. J., T. G. Ferris, and T. H. Lee. 2008. Options for slowing the growth of health care costs. *New England Journal of Medicine* 358(14):1509-1514.

Moses, H. 3rd, D. H. Matheson, E. R. Dorsey, B. P. George, D. Sadoff, and S. Yoshimura. 2013. The anatomy of health care in the United States. *JAMA* 310(18):1947-1963.

Moses, H. 3rd, D. H. Matheson, S. Cairns-Smith, B. P. George, C. Palish, and E. R. Dorsey. 2015. The anatomy of medical research: US and international comparisons. *JAMA* 313(2):174-189.

Pittman, P. 2010. Health services research in 2020: data and method needs for the future. *Health Services Research* 45(5):1431-1441.

Ravindranath, M. 2018, April 27. CMS to make Medicare Advantage data available to researchers. Politico. Retrieved from: https://www.politico.com/newsletters/morning-ehealth/2018/04/27/cms-to-make-medicare-advantage-data-available-to-researchers-190036.

Robinson, J. C., and T. T. Brown. 2013. Increases in consumer cost sharing redirect patient volumes and reduce hospital prices for orthopedic surgery. *Health Affairs* 32(8):1392-1397.

Sarnak, D. O., D. Squires, G. Kuzmak, and S. Bishop. 2017. *Paying for Prescription Drugs Around the World: Why Is the U.S. an Outlier?* The Commonwealth Fund.

Semmelweis, I. 1983. Etiology, concept, and prophylaxis of childbed fever. In: Carter KC, editor. 1st ed. Madison, WI: The University of Wisconsin Press.

Shah, S. P., L. McCourt, K. Jakobson, A. Saddington, K. Harvey, K. A. Schulman. 2018. Leading change—a national survey of chief innovation officers in health systems. *Health Management, Policy, and Innovation*, 3(1).

Siddons, A. 2018. Health Statistics See Funding Lag Amid Boosts Elsewhere. *Roll Call.*

Simpson, S. 2018. Show Me the Money! Trends in Funding for Health Services Research. *Health Services Research* (in press).

Song, Z., S. Rose, D. G. Safran, B. E. Landon, M. P. Day, and M. E. Chernew. 2014. Changes in health care spending and quality 4 years into global payment. *New England Journal of Medicine* 371(18)1704-1714.

Song, Z., S. Rose, M. E. Chernew, and D. G. Safran. 2017. Lower- versus higher-income populations in the Alternative Quality Contract: improved quality and similar spending. *Health Affairs* 36(1)74-82.

The SUPPORT Principal Investigators. 1995. A controlled trial to improve care for seriously ill hospitalized patients: the study to understand prognoses and preferences for outcomes and risks of treatments (SUPPORT). *JAMA* 274(20):1591-1598.

Tseng, P., R. S. Kaplan, B. D. Richman, M. A. Shah, and K. A. Schulman. 2018. Administrative Costs Associated With Physician Billing and Insurance-Related Activities at an Academic Health Care System. *JAMA* 319(7): 691–697.

U.S. Department of Health and Human Services. 2017. HHS FY 2017 Budget in Brief. https://www.hhs.gov/about/budget/fy2017/budget-in-brief/index.html. Accessed on November 2, 2018.

White, K. L., T. F. Williams, and B. G. Greenberg. 1961. The ecology of medical care. *New England Journal of Medicine* 265:885-892.

Appendix A:

BUILDING THE EVIDENCE BASE FOR IMPROVING HEALTH CARE PARTICIPANT LIST

MEETING PARTICIPANTS

Gerard F. Anderson, PhD
Director, Center for Hospital Finance
& Management
Johns Hopkins Bloomberg School of
Public Health

Mary Applegate, MD, FAAP, FACP
Medical Director
Ohio Department of Medicaid

Sharon B. Arnold, PhD
Deputy Director
Agency for Healthcare Research &
Quality

David Atkins, MD, MPH
Director, Health Services Research &
Development
US Department of Veterans Affairs

John Z. Ayanian, MD, MPP
Director, Institute for Healthcare
Policy & Innovation
University of Michigan

Alan Balch, PhD, MS
Chief Executive Officer
Patient Advocate Foundation

Richard A. Bankowitz, MD, MS,
MBA, FACP
Chief Medical Officer
America's Health Insurance Plans

Matt Barry, MPA
Section Research Manager
Congressional Research Service

Andrew Bazemore, MD, MPH
Director
Robert Graham Center

Anne Beal, MD, MPH
Chief Patient Officer & Global Head,
Patient Solution
Sanofi

Richard E. Besser, MD
President & Chief Executive Officer
Robert Wood Johnson Foundation

Karl Y. Bilimoria, MD, MS
John Benjamin Murphy Professor of
 Surgery
Northwestern University Feinberg
 School of Medicine

Leah Binder, MA
President & Chief Executive Officer
The Leapfrog Group

Andrew Bindman, MD
Professor of Medicine, Health Policy,
 Epidemiology & Biostatistics
University of California, San Francisco

David Blumenthal, MD, MPP
President & Chief Executive Officer
The Commonwealth Fund

William A. Bornstein, MD, PhD
Chief Medical Officer; Chief Quality
 & Patient Safety Officer
Emory Healthcare

Niall Brennan, MPP
President & CEO
Health Care Cost Institute

Craig Burns, PhD MS
Vice President of Research, Center for
 Policy & Research
America's Health Insurance Plans

Ann H. Cary, PhD, MPH, RN,
 FNAP, FAAN
Dean, School of Nursing and Health
 Studies
University of Missouri Kansas City

Tammy Chang, MD, MPH, MS
Assistant Professor, Department of
 Family Medicine
University of Michigan

Michael E. Chernew, PhD
Leonard D. Schaeffer Professor of
 Health Care Policy
Harvard Medical School

Carolyn Clancy, MD, MACP
Executive in Charge, Veterans Health
 Administration
US Department of Veterans Affairs

Eleanor Dehoney, MPH
Vice President, Policy and Advocacy
Research!America

Sanjay Doddamani, MD, FASE,
 FACC, FACP
Senior Director, Population Health
Geisinger Health System

Adaeze Enekwechi, PhD, MPP
Vice President
McDermott+Consulting

Timothy G. Ferris, MD, MPH
Chief Executive Officer
Massachusetts General Physicians
 Organization

Lee A. Fleisher, MD
Chair, Department of Anesthesiology
 & Critical Care
University of Pennsylvania Perelman
 School of Medicine

Sandro Galea, MD, DrPH
Dean
Boston University School of Public
  Health

Clif Gaus, ScD, MHA
President & Chief Executive Officer
National Association of ACOs

Atul Grover, MD, PhD
Executive Vice President
Association of American Medical
  Colleges

Kevin Grumbach, MD
Chair, Department of Family &
  Community Medicine
University of California, San Francisco

Emily J. Holubowich, MPP
Senior Vice President
CRD Associates

Charles N. Kahn III, MPH
President & Chief Executive Officer
Federation of American Hospitals

Gary S. Kaplan, MD, FACP, FACMPE,
  FACPE
Chairman & Chief Executive Officer
Virginia Mason Health System

Rainu Kaushal, MD, MPH
Chair, Healthcare Policy & Research
Weill Cornell Medicine

Gopal Khanna, MBA
Director
Agency for Healthcare Research and
  Quality

Shari M. Ling, MD
Deputy Chief Medical Officer
Centers for Medicare & Medicaid
  Services

Sean C. Lucan, MD, MPH, MS
Physician
Montefiore Medical Center

Andrew Lyzenga, MPP
Senior Director, Quality Measurement
National Quality Forum

Katie Martin, MPA
Vice President, Health Policy &
  Programs
National Partnership for Women &
  Families

George A. Mensah, MD
Director, Center for Translation
  Research & Implementation Science
National Heart, Lung, & Blood
  Institute
National Institutes of Health

Arnold S. Milstein, MD, MPH
Director, Clinical Excellence Research
  Center
Stanford University

Suzanne Miyamoto, PhD, RN, FAAN
Chief Policy Officer
American Association of Colleges of
Nursing

Alexander Ommaya, DSc
Senior Director, Clinical &
Translational Research & Policy
Association of American Medical
Colleges

Frank G. Opelka, MD
Medical Director
American College of Surgeons

Stephen T. Parente, PhD, MPH, MS
Professor
University of Minnesota

Mark V. Pauly, PhD
Professor, Health Care Management
Wharton School, University of
Pennsylvania

Eleanor M. Perfetto, PhD, MS
Senior Vice President, Strategic
Initiatives
National Health Council

Jonathan B. Perlin, MD, PhD, MSHA,
MACP, FACMI
President, Clinical Services & Chief
Medical Officer
Hospital Corporation of America

Robert Phillips, MD, MSPH
Vice President, Research & Policy
American Board of Family Medicine

Alonzo L. Plough, PhD, MA, MPH
Vice President, Research-Evaluation-
Learning & Chief Science Officer
Robert Wood Johnson Foundation

Tannaz Rasouli, MPH
Senior Director, Public Policy &
Strategic Outreach
Association of American Medical
Colleges

Erin Richardson, JD
Vice President & Associate General
Counsel
Federation of American Hospitals

Emily Roesing, MBA
Director, Business Development
Catalyst for Payment Reform

Kristin Rosengren
Vice President, Strategic
Communications
AcademyHealth

Meredith B. Rosenthal, PhD
Professor of Health Economics &
Policy
Harvard TH Chan School of Public
Health

Dana G. Safran, MA, ScD
Chief Performance Measurement
& Improvement Officer; Sr. Vice
President, Enterprise Analytics
Blue Cross Blue Shield of Massachusetts

Claudia Salzberg, PhD
Senior Vice President of Quality
Federation of American Hospitals

Darshak Sanghavi, MD
Chief Medical Officer & Senior Vice
  President of Translation
OptumLabs

Lewis G. Sandy, MD, MBA, FACP
Executive Vice President, Clinical
  Advancement
UnitedHealth Group

Lucy A. Savitz, PhD, MBA
Vice President, Health Research
Kaiser Permanente, Northwest Region

Kevin A. Schulman, MD, MBA
Professor of Medicine
Duke University

Joe V. Selby, MD, MPH
Executive Director
Patient Centered Outcomes Research
  Institute

Andrew Shin, JD, MPH
Chief Operating Officer, Health
  Research & Educational Trust
American Hospital Association

Lisa Simpson, MB, BCh, MPH, FAAP
President & Chief Executive Officer
  AcademyHealth

Julie Sochalski, PhD, RN, FAAN
Associate Dean for Academic Programs
University of Pennsylvania School of
  Nursing

Lina Walker, PhD
Vice President of Health Security
AARP Public Policy Institute

Jay Want, MD
Chief Executive Officer
Peterson Center on Healthcare

Alan Weil, JD, MPP
Editor-in-Chief
Health Affairs

Jack Westfall, MD, MPH
Director, Whole Person Care
Santa Clara Valley Medical Center

Modena Wilson, MD, MPH
Senior Vice President, Chief Health &
  Science Officer
American Medical Association

NAM Staff

Sameer Siddiqi
Technical Consultant

Urooj Fatima
Senior Program Assistant

Gwen Hughes
Research Coordinator

Danielle Whicher, PhD, MHS
Senior Program Officer

Michael McGinnis, MD, MPP
Executive Director, Leadership
    Consortium for a Value & Science-
    Driven Health System
Leonard D. Schaeffer Executive Officer

Appendix B:

BUILDING THE EVIDENCE BASE FOR IMPROVING HEALTH CARE SYMPOSIUM AGENDA

BUILDING THE EVIDENCE BASE FOR IMPROVING HEALTH CARE
Contributions, opportunities, and priorities

A NATIONAL ACADEMY OF MEDICINE SYMPOSIUM

February 26-27, 2018
National Academy of Sciences Building
Lecture Room
2101 Constitution Avenue NW
Washington, DC 20001

NAM Leadership Consortium for a Value & Science-Driven Health System

Meeting focus: Contributions of health services research (HSR) to effectiveness and efficiency in health and health care, and key priorities for HSR as a means of generating the evidence required to guide transformative progress in the next two decades.

Core questions
1. **Contributions:** How has HSR contributed to improvement in health gains and health care access, delivery, and quality—at various levels: system, organization, practice, and health–health care interfaces?
2. **Priorities:** What are the challenges, opportunities, and priorities for HSR in the next decade, and beyond, for improving access, safety, quality, value,

and patient/family engagement in a changing health care environment, while reducing spending growth and advancing population health progress?

3. **Support:** What are the current public and private sources of support for HSR, what trends are in play, and do the metrics of decision-making and assessment vary by source and focus (e.g., technology assessment, clinical guidelines, care quality and safety, primary care, utilization and financing)? What should be the role of federal funding for HSR, now and in the long-term?

4. **Organization:** How are HSR opportunities identified? How is HSR funded, coordinated, and results disseminated? How might these processes be improved? What is or should be the profile of a governance structure for HSR?

5. **Statutory mandate:** What might be the consequences if current legislative mandates related to HSR priorities—(e.g., a Center on Primary Care Research and the Centers for Education and Research on Therapeutics [CERTS])—were eliminated? How might important emphases be sustained and nurtured?

6. **Intended outcomes:** Identify unique opportunities for the field of HSR to advance rigorous, timely, and relevant evidence, and inform national progress toward a health system that is person-centered, high performing, and continuously learning.

DAY 1

8:30 AM   Coffee and light breakfast available

9:00 AM   Welcome and meeting overview

Welcome
  Michael McGinnis, National Academy of Medicine

Opening remarks
  Victor Dzau, National Academy of Medicine
  Lisa Simpson, AcademyHealth

9:30 AM   Health services research: field and impact to date

Focus: The nature of, and contributions from, health services research over the past two decades and its impact on health policy, health delivery systems, and health care efficiency and access.

David Blumenthal, The Commonwealth Fund
Leah Binder, The Leapfrog Group
Tim Ferris, Massachusetts General Physicians Organization

Q&A and Open Discussion

10:35 AM   Break

10:45 AM   Pressing issues and data infrastructure needs in health services research

Focus: The state of current compelling issues impacting quality, value, and equity that require health services research insights; the data infrastructure required to accelerate these insights.

Moderator: *Adaeze Enekwechi,* McDermott+Consulting

Panelists:
Andrew Bazemore, Robert Graham Center
Karl Bilimoria, Northwestern Medicine
Niall Brennan, Health Care Cost Institute
Katie Martin, National Partnership for Women & Families

Q&A and Open Discussion: What are the areas in greatest need of new evidence or widespread implementation of existing evidence? What are the opportunities and challenges with the data infrastructure to support advances in these areas?

12:00 PM   Lunch

12:30 PM   Emerging approaches to improving access to care

Focus: Emerging change dynamics affecting access to care; implications for the field of HSR.

Moderator: *Alonzo Plough,* Robert Wood Johnson Foundation

Panelists:
Sandro Galea, Boston University School of Health: Social determinants of health

Jack Westfall, Santa Clara Valley Medical Center: Linking primary care and social community services

Michael Chernew, Harvard Medical School: Innovations in consumer driven care

Gerard Anderson, Johns Hopkins University: Tiered networks, volume, and access to complex care

Q&A and Open Discussion: How is HSR meaningfully contributing to addressing these issues?

1:40 PM   Break

1:50 PM   Emerging approaches to care quality and efficiency

Focus: Emerging change dynamics impacting care quality and efficiency; implications for the field of HSR.

Moderator: *Jay Want,* Peterson Center on Healthcare

Panelists:

Dana Safran, Blue Cross Blue Shield of Massachusetts: Changing provider incentives by moving from fee-for-services to population-health payment model

Gary Kaplan, Virginia Mason Health System: Health systems engineering to improve patient, family, and clinician experience and outcomes

Rainu Kaushal, Weill Cornell Medicine: Identifying and Predicting High Need, High Cost Patients

Kevin Schulman, Duke University: Innovation models in health care

Q&A and Open Discussion: How is HSR meaningfully contributing to addressing these issues? What are the current challenges with leveraging health data to support HSR in these areas?

3:00 PM   Break

3:10 PM   The health services research ecosystem

Focus: Stakeholders involved in actively supporting, conducting, and implementing HSR; their interactions.

Presenter: Overview of the different actors involved in funding, conducting, and disseminating and implementing the findings from HSR; the federal investment and the public interest in supporting this field of research.

Lisa Simpson, AcademyHealth

Key perspective reactor panel
   Moderator: *Atul Grover,* Association of American Medical Colleges

   Reactors:
   Gopal Khanna, Agency for Healthcare Research and Quality
   George Mensah, National Institutes of Health
   Joe Selby, Patient Centered Outcomes Research Institute
   Shari Ling, Centers for Medicare & Medicaid Services
   David Atkins, US Department of Veterans Affairs

Q&A and Open Discussion: What are the unique roles of the federal government and private foundations in supporting HSR?

4:30 PM   Closing remarks: Remaining challenges

Closing remarks will outline the remaining challenges for the field of HSR in preparation for the day 2 discussions.
   Carolyn Clancy, US Department of Veterans Affairs

Reception

End of day one

DAY 2

8:30 AM   Day 1 Summary and Overview of Day 2

Michael McGinnis, National Academy of Medicine

**9:00 AM   Health services research priorities ahead from the user
                  perspective**

Focus: Based on the impact to date, remaining gaps, and field dynamics, assess priorities for the next decade and relevant data needs.

Moderator: *Arnie Milstein,* Stanford University

Charles Kahn, Federation of American Hospitals
Mary Applegate, Ohio Department of Medicaid
William Bornstein, Emory Healthcare
Lina Walker, AARP

Q&A and Open Discussion

10:20 AM   Break

10:30 AM   Health services research moving forward: strategy and coordination

Focus: Strategy for engaging the opportunities and priorities including strengthening the case for public interest in supporting HSR through federal investments and ideas for coordinating efforts and ensuring appropriate governance.

Moderator: *Jonathan Perlin,* Hospital Corporation of America

Andrew Bindman, University of California San Francisco
Bob Phillips, American Board of Family Medicine
Lee Fleisher, University of Pennsylvania
Ellie Dehoney, Research!America

Q&A and Open Discussion

11:45 AM   The imperative

Presentation: The charge and charter for the field of HSR over the next two decades.

Richard Besser, Robert Wood Johnson Foundation

12:15 PM   Closing comments

12:30 PM   Adjourn

SUPPORT FOR THIS MEETING WAS PROVIDED BY:*

AcademyHealth
American Association of Colleges of Nursing
American Board of Family Medicine
American Society of Anesthesiologists
Association of American Medical Colleges
Federation of American Hospitals
Robert Wood Johnson Foundation

Planning Committee

Andrew Bindman, MD, University of California San Francisco
Carolyn Clancy, MD, MACP, US Department of Veterans Affairs
Ellie Dehoney, MPH, Research!America
Adaeze Enekwechi, PhD, MPP, McDermott+Consulting
Lee Fleisher, MD, University of Pennsylvania
Sherry Glied, MA, PhD, New York University
Atul Grover, MD, PhD, Association of American Medical Colleges
Sandra R. Hernández, MD, California Health Care Foundation
Charles N. Kahn III, MPH, Federation of American Hospitals
Gopal Khanna, MBA, Agency for Healthcare Research and Quality
Suzanne Miyamoto, PhD, RN, FAAN, American Association of Colleges of Nursing
Robert Phillips, MD, MSPH, American Board of Family Medicine
Alonzo Plough, Robert Wood Johnson Foundation
Joe V. Selby, MD, MPH, Patient Centered Outcomes Research Institute
Lisa Simpson, MB, BCh, MPH, FAAP, AcademyHealth

* *The views expressed in the meeting and subsequent NAM Meeting Summary do not necessarily reflect the views of the National Academy of Medicine, the meeting planning committee, or funding organizations.*

CPSIA information can be obtained
at www.ICGtesting.com
Printed in the USA
BVHW091645080119
537259BV00006B/12/P